On the Politics of Ignorance in Nursing and Healthcare

T0372533

Ignorance is mostly framed as a void, a gap to be filled with appropriate knowledge. In nursing and healthcare, concerns about ignorance fuel searches for knowledge expected to bring certainty to care provision, preventing risk, accidents or mistakes. This unique volume turns the focus on ignorance as something productive in itself, and works to understand how ignorance and its operations shape what we do and do not know.

Focusing explicitly on nursing practice and its organisation within contemporary health settings, Amélie Perron and Trudy Rudge draw on contemporary interdisciplinary debates to discuss social processes informed by ignorance, ignorance's temporal and spatial boundaries, and how ignorance defines what can be known by specific groups with differential access to power and social status. Using feminist, postcolonial and historical analyses, this book challenges dominant conceptualisations and discusses a range of 'non-knowledges' in nursing and health work, including uncertainty, abjection, denial, deceit and taboo. It also explores the way dominant research and managerial practices perpetuate ignorance in healthcare organisations.

In health contexts, productive forms of ignorance can help to future-proof understandings about the management of healthy/sick bodies and those caring for them. Linking these considerations to nurses' approaches to challenges in practice, this book helps to unpack the power situated in the use of ignorance, and pays special attention to what is safe or unsafe to know, from both individual and organisational perspectives.

On the Politics of Ignorance in Nursing and Healthcare is an innovative read for all students and researchers in nursing and the health sciences interested in understanding more about transactions between epistemologies, knowledge-building practices and research in the health domain. It will also be of interest to scholars involved in the interdisciplinary study of ignorance.

Amélie Perron is Associate Professor in the School of Nursing, Faculty of Health Sciences, University of Ottawa, Canada.

Trudy Rudge is the Professor of Nursing (Social Sciences and Humanities) at Sydney Nursing School, University of Sydney, Australia.

Routledge Key Themes in Health and Society

Available titles include:

Turning Troubles into Problems
Clientization in human services
Edited by Jaber F. Gubrium and Margaretha Järvinen

Compassionate Communities
Case studies from Britain and Europe
Edited by Klaus Wegleitner, Katharina Heimerl & Allan Kellehear

Exploring Evidence-based Practice
Debates and challenges in nursing
Edited by Martin Lipscomb

On the Politics of Ignorance in Nursing and Healthcare
Knowing ignorance
Amélie Perron and Trudy Rudge

Forthcoming titles include:

Empowerment
A critique
Kenneth McLaughlin

Living with Mental Disorder
Insights from qualitative research
Jacqueline Corcoran

On the Politics of Ignorance in Nursing and Healthcare

Knowing ignorance

Amélie Perron and Trudy Rudge

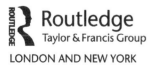

Routledge
Taylor & Francis Group

LONDON AND NEW YORK

First published 2016 by Routledge

2 Park Square, Milton Park, Abingdon, Oxon OX14 4RN
711 Third Avenue, New York, NY 10017, USA

Routledge is an imprint of the Taylor & Francis Group, an informa business

First issued in paperback 2017

British Library Cataloguing in Publication Data
A catalogue record for this book is available from the British Library

Library of Congress Cataloging in Publication Data
Perron, Amélie, author.
On the politics of ignorance in nursing and healthcare : knowing ignorance /
Amélie Perron and Trudy Rudge.
p. ; cm. -- (Routledge key themes in health and society)
Includes bibliographical references and index.
I. Rudge, Trudy, author. II. Title. III. Series: Routledge key themes in
health and society.
[DNLM: 1. Nursing. 2. Politics. WY 16.1]
RT41
610.73--dc23
2015008183

ISBN: 978-1-138-81966-5 (hbk)
ISBN: 978-1-138-63232-5 (pbk)

Typeset in Times New Roman
by Taylor & Francis Books

The certainty of incoherence in reading, the inevitable crumbling of the soundest constructions, is the deep truth of books. Since appearance constitutes a limit, what truly exists is a dissolution into common opacity rather than a development of lucid thinking. The apparent unchangingness of books is deceptive: each book is also the sum of the misunderstandings it occasions.

Georges Bataille, *The Bataille Reader* (Botting, F. and S. Wilson. (1997). *The Bataille Reader*. Oxford: Wiley-Blackwell.)

'Perron and Rudge provide an indispensable and clearly articulated work that situates the concept of ignorance in its rightful place as knowledge. The remarkable notion that nurses and others in health care pay attention to what is unknown, silenced, hidden, glossed over, and simply ignored should become an essential—a foundation to practice that is rooted in critical analysis. This is an important book as we head further into the 21st century, where the recognition and acknowledgement of what we do not know may be just the thing that saves humans and the planet. *On the Politics of Ignorance in Nursing and Health Care* is imperative reading to underpin the framework of any pedagogical, scholarly, clinical, administrative, or activist endeavor.'

Paula N. Kagan, PhD, RN, Associate Professor, School of Nursing, DePaul University Chicago, USA

Editor, Philosophies and Practices of Emancipatory Nursing: Social Justice as Praxis, *Routledge, 2014 (with Marlaine C. Smith and Peggy L. Chinn)*

'Perron and Rudge have delivered a provocative and original work. Shining a light on the darkness of ignorance, the authors reveal its uses and its political power in health care policy and practice. An intelligent and penetrating piece of scholarship, this is a book to unsettle the reader's certainties. Be prepared to embrace an ethics of discomfort!'

Sioban Nelson, Professor, Vice-Provost Academic Programs, Vice-Provost Faculty and Academic Life, University of Toronto, Canada

Contents

Acknowledgments

We wish to acknowledge all those nurses who 'know', whether intuitively, empirically or experientially, and whose knowledge continues to be resisted and ignored.

We would also like to acknowledge participants and colleagues who provided feedback and wide-ranging discussions about ignorance in all its forms.

We would like especially to acknowledge our colleagues Sandra West and Virginia Mapedzahama, who were our first collaborators on these matters;[1] participants at the Philosophy in the Nurses' World, Banff, Canada May 25–27, 2014, where Trudy Rudge presented on 'What has ignorance got to do with it?'; and Colleen Varcoe and the participants at the CRiHHI Critical Inquiry series, Nursing School, UBC, Vancouver, Canada—thank you for your interest and feedback about a paper entitled 'White ignorance: A lens to "explore" settler societies and discredited knowledge(s)'.

1 This is part of a research project on black migrant nurses: Mapedzahama, V., T. Rudge, S. West and A. Perron (2011). 'The unknowing 'other' or un/knowing the 'other'? Theorising ignorance and the maintenance of white privilege in Australian nursing workplaces.' New Orleans, 6th International Conference on Interdisciplinary Social Sciences.

1 Introduction

> It is a common sentence that Knowledge is power; but who hath duly considered or set forth the power of Ignorance?
>
> George Eliot, *Daniel Deronda,* 1876

> Up to this time in the history of man there has, with few exceptions, been an infatuated pursuit of this will-o'-the wisp, knowledge. Why should not man now turn his glance to ignorance, if it were only for a little while and for the sake of fair play?
>
> Richard Dowling, *Ignorant Essays,* 1858

These two quotes, published twenty years apart during the nineteenth century, provide an interesting starting point for our introduction because both indicate a rupture with the dominance of knowledge as the only way to 'know'. They also suggest a view of ignorance as something worthy of thinking and exploration, if only for balance and 'fairness'. It is our contention that with this book, we answer both Eliot's and Dowling's appeals.

Since the mid-1980s there has been increased interest in the idea of ignorance, not merely as knowledge's opposite, or as its absence in terms of the utilitarian view of knowledge, but increasingly as a concept that is in dynamic relation with knowledge, each mutually implicated in the production, reproduction and construction of what we know and do not know. Moreover, the concept of ignorance is viewed as having its own rules, epistemologies and sociology, implicated in knowledge production yet often using very different forms of production (Tuana 2006; Smithson 2008; Proctor and Schiebinger 2008; McGoey 2012a). For instance, Smithson notes that ignorance 'is an essential component in social relations, organisations and cultures. People are motivated to create and maintain ignorance, often systematically' (2008: 209). From such a view, ignorance is contrived through taking positions that define one as not knowing or unknowing, and there is some socio-political utility to maintaining or producing such a positioning.

Authors such as Tuana (2006), Smithson (2008) and McGoey (2012a) have asserted that there are taxonomies or epistemologies of ignorance that provide ways to understand how power and ignorance interact, how knowledge and ignorance intersect, and how ignorance is actively produced by the very practices that seek to uncover, expose and develop knowledge. As McGoey (2012a: 3) suggests, the study of produced and maintained ignorance is the search for knowledge's twin, not its opposite; as she puts this more simply, 'Ignorance *is* knowledge' (McGoey 2012a: 4, emphasis in original). Or as Gross (2007: 748) contends, 'non-knowledge or ignorance refers to a realm that escapes recognition'. McGoey develops a taxonomy of ignorance that is nuanced, showing how its variety leads to difference within any epistemic community. She outlines how ignorance can be thought of as emancipation, in that not knowing is freeing of responsibility; as the knowing that welcomes blindness, such as the well known closet of non-knowing about sexuality, or other forms of deliberate ambiguity as a refusal to be located or categorised; as a commodity (like its twin 'knowledge'), where there is gain, cost, benefit to 'failing to identify solutions to problems they purport [to be] unsolvable' (McGoey 2012a: 7); as a location inhabited by climate-change deniers, tobacco companies and big pharma companies; or as pedagogy—that is, where ignorance has the ability to teach us. She also uses the expression *strategic ignorance*, where ignorance meets the means of a government, organisation or individual (see also Bailey 2007). It is these acts of mis- or non-recognition with which this book is concerned most particularly, and how the potential for it ensures the production of ignorance and its effects in nursing and healthcare practices.

This book begins with the premise that ignorance has its own dynamics that run alongside other knowledge systems and perhaps even its own claims to truth—where ignorance is productive—that is, it produces its own set of activities. In this chapter we provide an outline of the general thinking about ignorance—epistemologies, sociology and pedagogies. We outline the argument that follows in the book about different aspects of ignorance, how it plays out in nursing and healthcare work, and its positive as well as its negative outcomes for nurses and other healthcare workers. Our primary focus is on nursing, but in many cases what plays out for nurses is common to many other professional groups in healthcare, as relations between the structures of ignorance and its epistemologies produce nursing and other healthcare research, educational imperatives and practices in the clinic.

When things go wrong with the flow of knowledge

> Knowledge ... is not itself power, although it is the magnetic field of power. Ignorance and opacity collude or compete with knowledge in mobilizing the flows of energy, desire, goods, meanings, persons.
>
> (Sedgwick 2008: 4)

The Winnipeg case

Between March 15 and December 21 1994, twelve children died while undergoing or shortly after having undergone cardiac surgery at a major hospital in

Winnipeg, Canada. The deaths occurred at the hands of an inexperienced surgeon, Dr Jonah Odim. Odim's surgical skills were not assessed prior to hiring. Yet he had never undertaken, without supervision, the challenging surgical procedures he was about to perform. Throughout 1994, numerous concerns were expressed about the number of errors, procedural anomalies and the surgeon's competence, and complaints were lodged by nursing and medical staff. Following the death of the twelfth child, the programme was shut down and an external review was commissioned. Parents learned about these issues only when the results of the external review, released in February 1995, led to the suspension of the programme and the issuing of a press release. An inquest, chaired by Judge Murray Sinclair, was instigated.

The Sinclair Report (Sinclair, 2000) identified several issues that contributed directly or indirectly to the death of the children, including recruitment practices at the facility, systemic communication problems, inadequate handling of complaints, staffing problems, poor treatment of nurses and the parents whose child had died, the lack of monitoring, and the fallibility of humans who can and do make mistakes. The report outlined thirty-six recommendations targeting the institution, the College of Physicians and Surgeons of Manitoba, and the Province of Manitoba. The report was generally well received, though parents were overwhelmingly frustrated that no-one was held accountable or punished for the death of their children. In professional and academic circles, the dramatic events led to numerous analyses of various aspects of the matter, such as the maintenance of professional competence, human factors and risk management, quality assurance, patient safety, the ethics of whistleblowing, and so on.

The Bundaberg case

In 2005, a Royal Commission[1] began in Queensland, Australia, investigating the work of Jayant Patel, employed as director of general surgery at Bundaberg hospital. This Commission was set up by the government of Queensland into its own healthcare system and the issues surrounding the regulation of medical practice by overseas trained doctors. This doctor was believed to have been involved in the deaths, which went unremarked, of ninety patients between 2003 and 2005 (Moreton 2005). A nurse, Toni Hoffman, nurse unit manager of the Intensive Care Unit at the hospital, had disclosed her concerns to management, without effect. She then turned to her local member of the state government to apply pressure external to the organisation as well as through a journalist in a major newspaper. Patel was allowed to leave the country, but had to return to testify and explain the deaths and chronic conditions resulting from his practices. The legal cases were not able to prove the negligence cases beyond reasonable doubt. Patel had omitted to notify the Queensland Medical Board that his licence had been revoked in New York in 2001, and that he had limited licence at the time of his employment by Queensland Health. His registration was not investigated at the time of his registration to Queensland.

Papers about these events emanate from authors concerned with hospital safety and quality with concerns over obvious failure to investigate the deaths and performance issues (Scott et al. 2008; Gluyas et al. 2011); failures of local administration and budget inadequacies to employ well qualified staff (Moreton 2005; The Lamp 2006; Scott et al. 2008); analysis of the legal case and the way commissions are set by government to attribute and distribute blame (Harvey and Faunce 2006; Prasser 2010); the ethics of whistle-blower protection (Johnstone 2011); and finally what to do in healthcare to prevent such tragedies from reoccurring (Moreton 2005; Scott et al. 2008; Gluyas et al. 2011).

The Mid Staffordshire NHS Foundation Trust (and the Francis Reports)

Following the survey of care in the Mid Staffordshire NHS Foundation Trust, UK, the Francis Reports of 2010 and 2013 were undertaken, leading to 'what was to become one of the worst scandals in the history of NHS' (Allen et al. 2013). The Public Inquiry followed the identification of a cluster of deaths. The details of the reports are not required here, but suffice to say that they generated a public outcry about nursing standards, with reports of failures of 'basic' care, unsafe delegation practices, and poor management of older persons with cognitive deficits. The two reports provide stories that are painful and shameful for nurses, or indeed any health professional, detailing how many patients' needs were neglected (Allen et al. 2013).

Responses to the reports have a tone of shocked disbelief that such a situation could occur. Yet, as Traynor (2014) recounts, there have been preceding failures, reports and scandals over the years. As Allen et al. (2013) point out, the NHS appears to be in a recursive cycle of past reviews and reports, with limited or ineffectual change. Rather, successive regimes of poor funding, inadequate staffing and under-resourcing became the norm. Analysts critique the organisation of care (Allen 2013; Latimer 2014); problems with nursing education (with university education thought to train nurses who are 'too posh to wash') and retention (with organisational practices forcing registered nurses away from the bedside) (Allen 2013; Traynor 2014; Latimer 2014); and the regulatory and governance structures of the NHS, which continues to fail the population despite the fondness and esteem in which the system is held (Hughes 2013). Butterworth (2014) condemns the way blame descends on the highly visible in the system, while managers remain hiding in plain sight.

Bauman (2001) notes how changes in politics of culpability that accompany the neorationalist effects on bureaucracy have led to blame being deflected away from politicians at the centre of parliamentary systems. As we can see from earlier vignettes of 'when things go wrong', seemingly modern, transparent and accountable organisations remain as arcane, stunted and secretive, with pathways as to who is accountable as murky as ever (Vaughan 1999)—some would say, deliberately so. Of note, and we return to this theme time and again throughout this book, is the 'interplay' between what is not known, unknown, and refused to be known (Gross 2007) around the explanations provided when things go wrong. Systemic failure (which these cases undoubtedly are) results in a foment of activity around policing, surveillance measures, and multiplication of calls for strategies—to improve lines of communication; to take seriously all members of the healthcare team; to make systems more transparent, accountable and safe by measuring, documenting and standardising protocols—all methodologies centrally undertaken in particular frameworks, all of which failed in the above cases. There are few explorations of what happens when only some issues are counted, or when knowledge is not transmitted, not disseminated, or robbed of its context—or how, as we come to understand, knowledge is always incomplete, partial (that is, biased), and contestable, and framed by a hard-won epistemic privilege so that much remains not known outside the parameters we have set to blind us. That is, we are made ignorant by our own epistemic practices (Code 2004; Sedgwick 2008; Townley 2011).

Ignorance: capturing its manifold articulations

> We live in an age of ignorance, and it is important to understand how this came to be and why… through mechanisms such as deliberate or inadvertent neglect, secrecy and suppression, document destruction, unquestioned tradition and myriad forms of inherent (or unavoidable) culturopolitical selectivity.
>
> (Proctor and Schiebinger 2008: vii)

Revisiting the Winnipeg, Bundaberg and Mid Staffordshire cases, this time through the lens of ignorance, we can paint different pictures—pictures that are not solely about professional competence, administrative procedures and quality assurance, but that highlight the epistemic arrangements allowing these events to unfold. For example, in examining the main issues identified by Sinclair (2000) in relation to the Winnipeg children, one can see how a number of them hinge on the improper flow of critical knowledge that could have saved most of the patients' lives. The negligent and casual manner in which information was (not) collected regarding Odim's competence; hazy lines of authority and lack of responsibility preventing the communication of concerns and implementation of safeguards; the treatment of nurses, whose 'subservient position' (Sinclair 2000: 477) and status as 'undertrained subordinates' (466) helped depict them as unpersuasive, distraught and emotional women (Sinclair 2000; Ceci 2004); the way parents of deceased children, and children to be recruited for surgery, were kept in ignorance of the unfolding crisis, raising questions about whether they had, in fact, provided 'fully informed consent' for the procedures; and the management of errors, near-miss events and critical incidents ignored by administrators. Ignorance was a powerful mediator of the events of 1994 insofar as knowledge was not collected, communicated, recorded or accepted. This left significant unknowns 'intact', leading to systemic failure. Oversight, blunted communication, neglect, denial, dismissal, censorship and omission are various expressions of ignorance that sustained the conditions resulting in the children's deaths.

In healthcare organisations, where care is increasingly monitored and standardised, certain kinds of knowledge enjoy particular authority and legitimacy. This is the case, for example, for administrative knowledge, which leads to various rules, policies and codes; and (bio)medical knowledge, as primary arbiter of clinical practice. As Townley (2011: xviii) argues, 'knowledge that counts is that which is authorised by the proper institutions'. In health organisations, nurses appear to be perceived as unreliable knowers, evident in the way nurses have little influence on organisational decisions and institutional policy (Institute of Medicine 2010; Robert Wood Johnson Foundation 2010). Townley's (2011) notion of 'division of epistemic labour' is useful here, wherein certain individuals or groups are credited as having extended or sophisticated understanding of the 'real' issues. Nurses in the Winnipeg case clearly did not enjoy any measure of epistemic legitimacy in the face of other established knowers (physicians, administrators). The division of epistemic labour in this setting was tied to particular subject—and gendered—positions which did not include that of 'credible knowers' (Ceci 2004: 76), because of an emphasis on nurses' purported irrationality and feelings, rather than their competence and their legitimate observations.

Re-examining the Bundaberg through an ignorance perspective, the ongoing failures of local management to heed the nursing unit manager's warnings speak to being blinded through denial, an element highlighted in the reports of the commission. Management chose not to hear, even succeeding in getting one commission stopped (Prasser 2010). McGoey (2007) has termed this 'a will to ignorance' in bureaucracies where what must be known remains steadfastly unknown; this was compounded by Queensland Health's and the regulatory authorities' failure, upon registering Patel, to check information readily available, even on the internet (Prasser 2010). Prasser highlights how administrative and governmental processes such as Royal Commissions act to 'damp down concerns, promote stability without involving any commitment of resources or tangible benefits to citizens, allowing them to deal with the "politics" of the situation rather than the situation itself': they are, in effect, 'blame minimisers' (2010: 81).

In examining these particular cases, we suggest that Townley's (2011) concept of epistemic labour can be productively put to work, especially in understandinghow knowledge circulates, or not, between healthcare professionals, patients and the wider public. Disclosure of information, through formal policy or whistleblowing, situates the individual as an agent within a broader epistemic community, whose agency revolves around the countering of ignorance regarding systemic or individual practices as a matter of fairness and justice. According to Braaten (1990), epistemic agency unfolds in relation to an agent's social environment. She makes a case for the need for social environments to sustain virtuous traits in the epistemic agent, such as moral conduct, compassion and fairness. Social environments are where agents learn prevailing rules, norms and standards, and where they fine-tune their intellectual and relational skills (see Latimer and Munro 2015). However, alienating social environments can breed just the opposite: indifference, disengagement and denial of humanity, as well as enrolment and compliance, rather than resistance to harmful norms (Rudge 2013).

As regards the Mid Staffordshire facility, problematic flows of knowledge were also identified. A major conclusion of the Francis report revolved around strategies to enforce the circulation of knowledge through practices of transparency and candour. As a result, healthcare providers have become legally bound to disclose to patients errors and near-miss events, which, according to Francis, will naturally lead to more trust between patients and healthcare professionals. It therefore falls on frontline care providers to identify issues, communicate them to patients and make amends for them. One could argue that Francis' instruction will help healthcare organisations become better social environments (as per Braaten 1990). The duty of candour can indeed work to amplify visibility of potential issues and instigate their remediation toward safer, more humane care. However, we suggest that it could be equally obscuring: while it appears as supporting a culture of disclosure and learning from mistakes, it imbues nurses and other health professionals with the significant responsibility of transacting between healthcare organisations and patients, running the risk of presenting errors mainly as individual events, originating from a person or a group of persons whose competence or knowledge may appear as deficient. As Bauman (2001) highlights, a focus on individuals maintains ignorance about the ways organisational or broader systemic issues are at play in how errors or near misses occur. If we are to take Braaten's argument seriously, in considering nurses as epistemic, moral agents, we must account for the way their social environment enables or restricts their epistemic agency, and defines the value or the risk attached to particular knowledges that nurses come to handle through professional practice. While organisations such as the Nursing and Midwifery Council in the UK underscore nurses' duty of candour, they are less forthcoming regarding whether nurses, in reporting adverse events or near misses to patients, should disclose the systemic issues (e.g. enduring inadequate staffing ratios) fuelling these occurrences. Nurses handle various kinds of information that needs to be shared for legal, safety and moral reasons, but that may be perceived as too risky or cumbersome to disseminate. Here the importance of nurses' social environment plays out in powerful ways, possibly leading to organisational 'forgetting' (Rudge 2003).

One would think that defining ignorance would be easy and unproblematic, perhaps as absence of knowledge about something, someone, some action. However, as Matthias Gross (2007) points out, for each fact discovered there seems to be an exponential increase in our ignorance—how much this discovery has opened up for us to know. In such a ferment, the earlier quote by Proctor and Schiebinger (2008) begins to make sense. Moreover, there are twin paradoxes in operation here—first, that at a time when we appear to know so much, the limits to knowledge are more obvious; and second, that similarly it has become more difficult for us to define what is meant by knowledge, or indeed ignorance, as both slip away from our previous certainties about what each means in relation to each other.

Hence, this book is asking questions about the politics of ignorance in nursing and healthcare, and is located in the

> study of non-knowledge or the art of how knowledge is deflected, covered and obscured.... [Such] antiepistemology asks after its shadow: the nature of non-knowledge, and the political and social practices embedded in the effort to suppress or to kindle endless forms of ambiguity and ignorance.
>
> (McGoey 2012a: 3)

Code provides a strategic view of ignorance (strategic because linked to power relations) which is very useful to set out the politics of ignorance. Her 2004 paper entitled 'The power of ignorance' uses the work of James Mill and *The History of British India* where ignorance of the language, land and culture on the 'subcontinent' was conceived as a strength providing Mill with objectivity and useful distance with which to tell the story of British colonisation of India. One of the common hallmarks of colonisation is that settlement occurs under the condition of *terra nullius*, a self-proclaimed right to ignorance claimed through the pride and arrogance of a colonising power—'there was nothing here before us'—a form of mis- or non-recognition as ignorance. A further form of ignorance is represented by George Eliot's portrayal of Gwendolen Harleth in *Daniel Deronda* as ignorant of the 'very fact of her privilege, of the day to day constraints straitened circumstances entail, and of "other" lives lived daily in just such circumstances' (Code 2004: 291), where as an individual Gwendolen is 'ignorant of her own ignorance of everyday lives that are not hers' (294). In such portrayals, 'issues of culpability figure among the ethical epistemological questions posed by ignorance exposed, it is not easy to see how to weigh ignorant ignorance, morally, against conscious, self-congratulatory ignorance' (294). For Code, there is no space free of ignorance, pointing to 'the impotence of the epistemologies of mastery' (299) in answering the questions in front of us at this time.

Framework for questioning ignorance in nursing and health

An analysis of ignorance within nursing and healthcare must include a focus on both the individual and the institution. A person can be deemed to hold expert knowledge while another is not; a researcher may single-handedly decide which course of inquiry to pursue and which one to ignore. Through authority and discretion, each of these individuals is instrumental in controlling the production and the flux of information within a collective (clinical team, research institute, etc.). Conjuring the notion that individuals interact with a collective lends more weight still to Braaten's (1990) valuing of epistemic agents' social environments. Examining interactions between agents and the collective is a matter of epistemology and politics, because knowledge always entails power relationships and *vice versa* (Foucault 1977). Therefore, if one is sensitive to the role of institutions in knowledge production and circulation, one can be responsive to their function in the production and distribution of ignorance. While countless books and papers address issues of knowledge (and gaps in knowledge) in nursing and healthcare, none discusses the issue of ignorance as a concept in its own right. Here, ignorance is approached from a more productive and political (and, in some regards, more positive) perspective, a view that is rarely taken up in health-related fields. We contend that introducing the topic of ignorance in nursing and health scholarship is important because of its various, though often undetected, forms and its sustained effects—positive and negative, productive and detrimental—on care practices, health education, care administration and health research.

Feminist and postcolonial scholars have long delineated how systematic obfuscation and suppression of knowledge have led to the absence of certain voices and perspectives in research, public policy, healthcare and education. Yet this instrumental scholarship is not always acknowledged in 'ignorance studies', despite its clear anti-epistemological pitch. For example, in the introduction of a book co-edited with Londa Shiebinger, Robert Proctor (2008) falls into this trap by emphasising the novelty of ignorance studies (and suggesting new terminology for it) as though it has recently emerged as a fresh new field of inquiry. While prominent feminists such as Nancy Tuana and Londa Schiebinger appear in the collection, 'ignoring' the longstanding contribution of feminist and postcolonial scholars to, precisely, an epistemology of ignorance is remarkable. This is not to say that Proctor does not bring something to the field, but it does suggest how easy it is to discursively overlook, suspend, forget or obscure certain ideas. It also highlights the importance of engaging with the *idea* of ignorance from a variety of perspectives, even when the term 'ignorance' is not specifically used. This is where we begin.

In Chapter 2, using contemporary discussions in 'ignorance studies' and other disciplines, we explore how the concept of ignorance can be thought through and articulated in contexts where knowledge constitutes a dominant driver of (health) discourses, interventions and innovations; social processes informed by ignorance; how ignorance is set temporally and spatially; and how it defines who/what can be known by specific groups with differential access to power and social status. Critical perspectives, including feminist, postcolonial and historical analyses, are drawn upon to challenge dominant conceptualisations of ignorance. Rather than dissect the current literature according to disciplinary or theoretical allegiance, we choose to approach it according to various features of ignorance as proposed by Proctor: its history, its geography, its political economy and its morality. We believe this approach helps to engage multiple, interdisciplinary readings of ignorance in a less predictable manner.

In Chapter 3, we broaden the concept of ignorance to consider other types of 'non-knowledge' in nursing and health work, including uncertainty, confidentiality and deceit. Ignorance has a key role to play in our increasingly risk-averse society. For instance, in medical science much of what is considered 'ignorance' relates to what medical practitioners do not yet know, thus impeding accurate predictions of treatment outcomes, risks or management of uncertainties. Therefore, in health contexts, productive forms of ignorance help to future-proof understandings about the management of healthy/sick bodies and subjectivities. Here we problematise the dominant perception that science and rationality can provide definite answers to feelings of uncertainty, risk and vulnerability, and can sustain actions undertaken to relieve such unsettling states.

In Chapter 4, we pay special attention to the way ignorance underpins efforts to delineate what is safe or unsafe to know. In nursing, various subject matters remain taboo, unspoken and therefore unknown, which works to exclude certain discourses, experiences, knowledges, and even subjects. Nursing practice often takes place in areas where there exist suppressed forms of knowledge. For instance, taboos are often portrayed as things best not known or discussed. Nurses and other health professionals also work with the abject: they must routinely cast aside everyday horrors such as traumatic injuries, intimate partner violence, death and dying, child abuse, and other 'betrayals' to their norms, values and expectations. Nurses must manage these experiences in ways that safeguard their ability to care for patients but also for themselves; this may include overlooking or avoiding certain demands or situations, while concealing feelings of fear or disgust. Ignorance deployed in this way plays a vital role as a strategy of self-preservation. 'Dangerous' knowledge in health work is a fundamental aspect of anti-epistemological analyses, yet it remains surprisingly overlooked in current scholarship, except perhaps as an object of bioethical deliberation.

In Chapter 5, the book turns more explicitly to the politics of ignorance, though this is addressed in various ways throughout the entire book. Just as there are politics of knowledge, there is a mirror version, the politics of ignorance, where ignorance can and must be strategically managed towards a particular goal. As Lorraine Code notes, there is power associated with ignorance as much as there is with knowledge. In this chapter, we steer the discussion towards ignorance as a feature of the management of life processes, explicitly linking it with matters of biopolitics. We use the example of influenza immunisation and treatment to explore the ways in which what is unknown or dismissed can be used to achieve specific, state-defined purposes. Discussing the (bio)politics of ignorance helps to move beyond negative views of ignorance by outlining its productive effects. Ignorance, then, cannot be considered as an unproblematic, symmetrical complement to knowledge. It engenders its own political economy and associated discourses and subjective experiences.

In Chapter 6, we examine how nurses mobilise knowledge and ignorance in various ways to support practice or manage ideological processes that suppress some forms of practice over others. For example, nurses' use of contemporary research practices such as evidence-based practice leads them to overlook other ways of acquiring knowledge about patient or nurse experiences. These research practices gloss over enduring uncertainties about patient care that remain unaddressed by the so-called gold standard of experimental research, the randomised controlled trial. By engaging with and mobilising various forms of ignorance, nurses reinforce the political nature of their professional work, when they are enrolled into the apparatus of evidence-based practice, knowledge utilisation and the audit culture, all-pervasive in the education, health and research industries. This complex apparatus produces within it a range of forms of ignorance that were originally designed to build nursing knowledge. Paradigmatic orthodoxy and singular approaches to knowledge-building produce knowledge that is of little relevance, and nurses develop resistance to using this non-knowledge. However, nurses as care organisers have been less resistant to the audit culture, which increasingly diverts nursing efforts away from nursing practice, towards the wellbeing of the system itself.

In closing, we offer a form of active ignorance, that is, empathic ignorance, in recognition of ignorance as relational (a relation between self and the Other) wherein what is not known is privileged. Such a view allows epistemic agency and trust in social relations, and overcomes various failings associated with unknowns. It offers a resistant positioning to those forms of ignorance that assume epistemic privilege, granting agency, and a strategic positionality where power/ignorance can minimise the effects of racism, gender discrimination, ethnocentrism or ageism.

Note

1 A Royal Commission is proclaimed by a government so as to obtain an independent judicial review of governmental practices, where the Commission has the right to interrogate those brought before the Commission under oath. This implies any failure to provide truthful evidence can result in a trial for perjury should such evidence be found to be untrue. In this case there were two reviews, with one stopped due to claims of bias accepted by the High Court of Queensland, then reopened with a new Commissioner and terms of reference (Prasser 2010).

2 Ignorance

Current conceptualisations

In nursing education, transferable skills are a particularly hot commodity. This is captured in the common, though not necessarily accurate, saying that 'a nurse is a nurse is a nurse', an expression that implies that all nurses share the same skills and knowledge, regardless of their area of practice and personal dispositions. Acquiring the proper competencies has been touted as a pivotal condition to safe and effective care—care that reduces the risk of complications, hospital stays and costs (Anema and McCoy 2010). It is also put forth as a must for the nursing profession toward the exercise of increased influence on policy matters. Because nurses play a most prominent role in healthcare provision, and because they are called upon to strengthen their involvement in the policy arena, they are said to be knowledge workers (Snyder-Halpern et al. 2001) with a clear role to play in the knowledge economy. This includes, for example, promoting collaborative partnerships, better articulating nursing's contribution or the nature of nursing knowledge, fostering a sense of curiosity and inquiry among nursing students and graduates, and promoting innovation while allowing mistakes (see e.g. Freshwater 2004; Myrick 2005). Moreover, the need for increased specialisation, discussed above, is particularly evident in healthcare, including in nursing. Knowledge and expertise are the hallmarks of specialisation, and yet can be considered as encouraging ignorance through the narrowing effects of specialist expertise and lack of contact with nurses across specialisations. As we saw in Chapter 1 of this book, ignorance surfaces in surprising and multiple ways.

There are challenges in summarising the extensive writing on ignorance in contemporary work on knowledge, and in agreement with Proctor (2008), we see that ignorance can be accorded a history, geography, political economy and even a morality ('what you don't tell others can't hurt them'; for example, nurses may withhold information from patients to avoid causing harm). It is temporally and spatially defined (slogans by businesses may claim that knowledge is now/the future; science for tomorrow; knowledge lives here; knowledge is global; better science/truth for better tomorrow, etc.). Existing literature in the social science and humanities disciplines explores these features in a similar manner, where ignorance is seen as influencing, and being influenced by, different disciplinary frameworks. Before we move on to apply ideas about ignorance in nursing and healthcare, we first need to sift through the burgeoning body of literature on ignorance. To do this, we propose to organise this complex literature according to the features outlined by Proctor.

Histories of ignorance

A common linking of ignorance to history occurs when commentators (e.g. Hume 1994; Shribman 2006; Jones 2012) suggest that today's children or citizens of particular countries are ignorant of their history, such ignorance meaning that without historical knowledge, citizens cannot make meaningful political or civic decisions. Of course, such a characterisation relates to 'every-one' having access to 'a' history of their country. However such a stance does not take into account the historical production and/or maintenance of ignor-ance through careful and systematic concealing, suppression, forgetting and discrediting of particular types of knowledges that threaten or effectively dis-rupt established ideas, discourses and practices. This means that what counts as a history that would dispel 'ignorance' when it is conceived of as a gap is never as simple as many commentators would suggest. Moreover as Foucault (1970) points out in *The Order of Things*, what we have as history is a history told by those who gained dominance, with losers' knowledge(s) being lost or diminished in the telling of history. Such a view is also promoted by feminists such as Sullivan and Tuana (2007) and many social and science historians (Ginzburg 1989; Schiebinger 2008; Magnússon 2010; Nozawa 2012), particu-larly those who apply micro-history techniques and historiographical practices that use evidence from texts such as diaries, letters and other documents from 'ordinary' people with everyday interests and lives. This leads to the view that all histories are only partial histories, always contested and contestable. The problem arises, therefore, when one history is called 'our history' over another.

Such blindness as historical ignorance has been an effective mechanism in the history of colonisation of non-Europe by Europe from the seventeenth century onwards. Revisions on histories of colonisation have revealed several forms of non-knowing, unknowing and discrediting of local knowledges held by Indigenous populations (Mayor 2008; Wylie 2008). These are effectively achieved through the suppression of fossils and artefacts from Indigenous societies, inadvertent neglect or conscious discrediting of Indigenous ways of knowing (e.g. Stenhouse 2005; Proctor and Schiebinger 2008; Gammage 2012; Owen 2012). All of these processes became part of colonisation, and uncovering of this knowledge is central in postcolonial analyses where such knowledges are shown to be strategic ignorance that sustained the power relations of colonisation (Owen 2012), and legitimated ongoing removal of resources and prospecting of natural and mineral resources under advanced global capitalism.

As colonisation occurred simultaneously with the development of Enlight-enment thinking and the growth of merchant political and economic power, a form of strategic ignorance came into play—one that was blind to the culture of the populations being colonised, and also the state of affairs of the country that was colonised for its resources, land and potential source of geopolitical power for the colonisers. Legitimising of the colonisers' actions took place through the ways in which the 'less' civilised were to be colonised, and was determined through the metropolitan centre's definition and characterisation of what could be thought of as 'civilised' (Harris 1995; Code 2004; Wolloch 2007). Collections of specimens retrieved by museums in colonising countries; publications of historical treatises, pamphlets and volumes about colonised countries; and books by experts and authoritative figures—such as James Mill (1773–1836) and Edward Gibbon (1737–1794) in the UK, Antoine-Yves Goguet (1716–1758) and Jean-Jacques Rousseau (1712–1778) in France—promoted a certain kind of history, based on a careful selection and description of events that generally promoted colonial powers and interests against the 'local' knowns of the colonised. For example, in James Mill's *History of British India* (1817, cited in Code 2004), in which he attacks the history, religion, literature, customs and laws of India as traditionalist rather than as representing an ancient culture, he discredits and diminishes a culture in order to first deface it in the name of legitimising what happened upon colonisation. His book was influential in shaping ideas about the colonising of India, but has had ongoing effects on contemporary representations about India that remained influential throughout the former British Empire (Code 2004). Indeed, as Lamont and Bates (2007: 310, citing Lewis Wurgaft 1983) assert, colonial relations both in India and in metropolitan UK rested on a 'sense of the "illusion" of British colonial rule, power that rested on "mutual make believe"'. All of this ignorance comes under what Edward Said (2003) characterised as Orientalism, most importantly about the Near East in his case, but which can equally apply to metropolitan ignorance about all colonies, sustained and reproduced to this day in the role that metropolitan power maintains in former colonies and the creative destruction that ensued from the organised forgetting since colonisation (see Giroux 2014).

Moreover, this sustained unknowing or ignorance is not just about the colonised South, but is sustained about marginalised groups in metropolitan societies, their internal displacements and migrations (Haebich 2011). For instance, geographical histories of Europe have begun to uncover what was covered up by Enlightenment views of knowledge and ignorance (see Siddle 1992), which constructed a particular middle class sensibility and set of values as dominant from that time onwards. He maintains that what was valued as knowledge, and who was considered ignorant, was located along the pathways of travel for this middle class, and it is difficult to ascribe to this a purely urban knowledge/rural ignorance dichotomy. Siddle asserts that to maintain this as so, is to deny the subtle shifts in what was known and not known in the spread of knowledge associated with the bourgeoisie in France at this time.

Education is a prime space to disseminate certain kinds of ideas and socialise students as to what can be known, by whom, about what. Education can therefore comprise historical (and contemporary) subjugation of women's ways of knowing and doing. Female authors and philosophers have a history, even up to contemporary times, of hiding their 'discredited' identity as women so as to publish their work (e.g. Louisa May Alcott, Charlotte and Emily Brontë, George Sand, Harper Lee, P.D. James, J.K. Rowling). Early feminists also called for open access to education to protect and emancipate women from their state of ignorance. This call was repeated in the second wave of feminism (Cook 2009), where ignorance was not only pinned to women but also to the unknowns about women perpetuated by patriarchal knowledge development practices (Code 1991; Alcoff 2007; Tuana 2008). However, this also affected women's knowledge, and what was known and understood as women's intellectual abilities depended on whether girls and women were accorded value in the face of male dominance as gender intersected with class, race and ethnicity (Alcoff and Potter 1993). Gaztambide-Fernandez (2012) asserts that curriculum pasts are embedded in present developments. He suggests that an example of effects in curriculum in the present is seen in how current knowledge about neuroscience is replicating the way eugenicist beliefs were taken up in purportedly progressive educational works such as those of John Dewey (1859–1952). Curricula today are captive to similar uncritical discourses—what Gaztambide-Fernandez terms neuromyths—about the way learning occurs in the mind through pictures of brain activity. Other historical thinking is embedded around ways to engage Indigenous peoples with the educational system. Settlers' unconscious white ignorance racialises the colonised Other, and leads to whiteness embedded in curricula that lead to failure to properly engage with Indigenous peoples (Hage 1998; Haebich 2011).

Geographies of ignorance

Separation of history and geography is difficult when exploration of the intersection between knowledge and ignorance is dealt with in each epistemic system—histories and geographies are intertwined. This is especially the case in analysing the geopolitical strategising of colonial powers and the management of what were designated as dangerous, unruly knowledges that were at odds with a 'scientific' view of the world, being used to realise colonial objectives (Hage 1998; Mills 2007; Moreton-Robinson 2009). In order to know the native Other, studies of 'mankind' were established. This form of knowledge (the science of the study of 'man') garnered knowledge about natives and about the cultures being colonised, interpreted by outsiders. Privileging dominant forms of knowledge such as those promoted by the Enlightenment and modernism of colonisation (Mair et al. 2012) often led to misinterpretations and discrediting of local knowledges. Such ignorance blended selective and strategic ignorance, now recognised as cultural and white ignorance—a form of explanation that is blind to ways in which ethnic and racialised 'not knowing' are operationalised (Hage 1998; Bailey 2007; Mills 2007). Moreover, such discursive positioning extends to how the north–south divide is discussed and analysed, either when developmentalism is to be critiqued, or when theories from the North are used to ignore the realities of development for the populations of the South (Simon 1998).

These ways of characterising (and running) the world are represented in assumptions contained by and centred on a eurocentric point of view (Lewis 2000). Moreover, such views do not take into account variations in cultural approaches as to what is and what is not appropriate in specific cultures (see Wylie 2008; Keighley 2012). Interrogating such forms of cultural ignorance problematises the homogenising forces resulting from globalisation, where some continents and their countries remain *terra incognito* despite the time and resources spent 'discovering' and knowing them (Binns 2007). Indeed, this failure to engage meaningfully with other cultures means that many assumptions are carried unreconstructed from one global location to another. From the point of view of those who use cultural (or white) ignorance to marginalise and to 'other', their ignorance continues the belief in natives or other cultures being unsophisticated and 'traditional' (Keighley 2012: 182); or in native ignorance (Smithson 2008).

Such operations are common in the geographies of education, where Westernised textbooks, curricula and pedagogical practices are distributed and used globally. Here, students/learners migrating from the 'developing' world to Western countries are accompanied by ideas that reproduce the immigrant or globalised student as ignorant. As Schely-Newman (2011) shows in her analysis of a literacy programme for immigrants to the state of Israel, who *is* ignorant can be destabilised if one interrogates the forms of 'ignorance' at play in such encounters.

> From the perspective of the Establishment, old ways of knowledge were considered ignorance, to be eradicated. Former teachers rejected the concept of ignorance; over and again, they assured me that their students were not ignorant but lacked specific skills. The teachers' narratives emphasised mutual learning: 'We eradicated our own ignorance.' The third version is that of the female students, who challenged the need to eradicate anything. Rather than replacing old modes of knowledge with new ones, they chose to add skills to their repertoire, tailored to their own needs.
>
> (Schely-Newman 2011: 28)

While the above forms of ignorance are predicated more on non-recognition of knowledge and ignorance due to location, knowledge production in the Western world has come to dominate globally as much as within each country's jurisdiction. The institutions that dominate the landscape of knowledge production consist of Western universities, global research institutes and funding bodies, and publication in scientific journals. Practices legitimised in these globalised institutions influence what counts as knowledge in neocolonialism where Westernised research practices are transported unproblematically into the developing world. Supposedly non-biased approaches to drug developments have a 'place' as a requirement to obtain global reach of randomised controlled trials (RCTs). Debates about the external validity of drug trials and RCTs began this critique, insisting on inclusion of women; they have extended to obtain the important drug-use approvals in the West. Drugs have to be tested in multiple locations with diverse populations. However, this brings with it such problems as normatively induced ignorance (Kleinman and Suryanarayanan 2012), and these failures in outcomes are magnified when relocated into other locations where local knowledge is often not recognised, or is discredited and marginalised.

Knowledge is also an instrument of colonialism, 'exporting' best practice guidelines, evidence-based practice, managerialist discourses and practices, or nursing theories to the 'developing' world. This often occurs in the guise of development programmes through the World Health Organization (WHO) or philanthropic and religious groups, bringing knowledges that take precedence over local and specific knowledges that are assumed to promote ignorance, while the knowledge promoted by such groups is seen as providing modern skills and lifestyles to countries in need. Globalising of risks, uncertainty and the seeming connectedness of everything have hastened the process of denial of jurisdictional geographic realities; the developing and developed world's futures are viewed as more linked into a contemporary world (Ruckert 2013). Furthermore, other forms of knowing about geography, which were considered reliable and valid ways to understand geographies through stabilised locations, are no longer useful ways to comprehend the destabilised world of transnational economies or permeable boundaries of the developing South. van Schendel (2002) argues that, alongside more traditional geographies or national boundaries and locales, we need to explore what is made invisible in holding with such constructions.

As in other social sciences, what counted as knowledge about geography in the twentieth century has developed a more nuanced account of space and place, calling for geographies that do not flatten difference, or localities that are important in understanding how geography (as space and place) affects human relationality (Thrift 2004; Duff 2010). Geographical knowledges turned to explore geographies of inclusion and also exclusion through modes of production and economies of containment and consumption of human capital in particular geographic locations (Siddle 1992; Sorenson 2003; Swan 2010). Falling within such analyses are ghettos, favelas and other situations entailing the disposal or dispersal of human populations (Bauman 2004, 2011); controls of migration and immigrant knowing (Siddle 1992); and racism and the white ignorance identified above in histories of ignorance (Greer 2004; Feenan 2007; Mills 2007; Yancy 2008).

Moreover, what counts as a spatial analysis has changed dramatically because what was previously seen as distant geographically has been made visible, through apparently increasing intimate relations encouraged by information networks, rapid travelling of news, and ease of travel. However, just as there are flows of information or knowledge about such instances, there are associated flows of ignorance. Such flows are organised via the actions of exclusion and inclusion in spaces both at the level of the global and at the level of place—a form of ignorance that works on locality or the spatial dynamics where subjectivity is formed in national jurisdiction, international intersection, or in the organisations where we all work (Landzelius 2009). As van Schendel notes:

> cartographic peripheralisation is indicative of marginal status of an area in area studies, not just in terms of physical distance to some imagined area core, but also in terms of perceived relevance to the main concerns and problematiques that animate the study of the area.
>
> (van Schendel 2002: 652)

Some of the ignorance explored above is played out in spaces where such dynamics are not apprehended through normative science (Bauman 2000), where differences are flattened as to how a place, a location may have completely different geographies or sense of space. Such failure to recognise differences leads to the trivialisation of the distinctiveness of the place, rendering it insignificant (see Ahmed 2008; Tantchou 2014). Harrison (2000) highlights how understanding human everyday activities is difficult because of their ephemeral nature: transient behaviours that may or may not be recorded in their location, but that contribute to people's understanding of space, its emotionality as well as how place comes to be remembered, forgotten or ignored as central to human relations.

Dodge and Kitchin (2013) highlight that, in networks and flows of knowledge, different forms of unknowns play out in web-based information economies. In an analysis of prosumerism (mixed with older forms of capitalist production), they examine use of metadata and forms of mapping (sometimes knowingly by consumers), often in ignorance as to what happens to this information, provided willingly in the name of proactive choice by active consumers. And finally, Landzelius (2009) suggests that power, knowledge and space interact, intersect and are constitutive of how geographies and their memories are elaborated. Spatial configurations of forgetfulness–ignorance–power constitute subjectivities and social relations under advanced capitalism. Ignorance and forgetfulness are crucial, Landzelius asserts, to the reification and alienation of space in the political economy of capitalism.

The political economy of ignorance

Discussing the histories and geographies of ignorance clearly involves an examination of the way individuals and populations have organised themselves and their activities over time and in multiple spatial and social distributions. Economic growth is a powerful driver of the planning, implementing and evaluating of economic activities and performance. Ignorance is very much part of this process, though it is generally associated with the unpredictability of complex market and price systems that are organised in far-reaching network interactions. Economic uncertainty encourages the search for knowledge, and its role in the configuration of economic relations is undeniable. The link between knowledge—especially scientific knowledge—and economies has been clearly established by influential authors such as Kuznets, who argued that

> *all* empirical knowledge, all scientifically tested information, no matter how abstract and remote it may seem, is potentially applicable in economic production. Science, no matter how abstruse, is analysis of the world around us, and economic production is one type of manipulation of this world […] All empirical knowledge is thus potentially relevant to economic production.
>
> (Kuznets 1968: 61, emphasis in original)

Given the complexity of economic systems and the wide variety of actors that play a part in them, knowledge must come from a variety of sources, including mathematics, natural history, engineering, geography, biology (e.g. agronomy), health-related or medical knowledge, sociology and informatics, to name a few. Useful, practical knowledge, then, is understood as the source of modern economic growth.

This has led to what is termed the *knowledge economy*, an economic structure in which advanced economies rely on activities and entities that become more and more abstract. Over the past decades, according to various economic authorities, tangible entities such as natural resources, human labour and physical capital have lost their privileged position as the main inputs of economic activity. In most post-industrial, advanced economy nations, the knowledge economy has effectively replaced agriculture-, industry- and service-based economies, inasmuch as knowledge, rather than farming, manufacturing or human labour, becomes a prime economic good. The core notion of the knowledge economy is the exchange of knowledge, in much the same way as any other commodity or resource used in various types of economic activity in order to generate wealth. The concept is tightly linked with other concepts, including knowledge user, knowledge society, knowledge workforce, knowledge mobilisation, knowledge-based firms, and human capital. A knowledge society, for example, can be understood as one that is built and organised around the creation and the use of knowledge so as to ensure the social and economic development of society. The role of technology in this process is fundamental, but, as expected, so too is the role of scientific research and education infrastructures, which work to produce knowledge as well as impart and apply knowledge.

Within the neoliberal mindset, knowledge development and dissemination are therefore highly contextual, the result of innovation-driven research that is expected to lead to new business opportunities, new products and new trades. They must therefore be highly responsive to shifting socioeconomic developments and demands, such as the proliferation of technology in all aspects of life, the globalisation of the workforce, and changing regional, national and world demographics. These notions provide very utilitarian and pragmatic views of knowledge and its role in society. They also lead to particular understandings of what kind of knowledge is needed (valued) to sustain the economy; who is 'knowledgeable'; and how knowledge should be imparted. Education, for instance, is seen as one of the most salient features and supports of a knowledge economy, insofar as it is explicitly tied to labour market needs and priorities. Particular educational approaches, such as problem-based learning and competency-based education, which are said to provide learners with practical skills for the real world, inscribe themselves within a discourse of education as something that must support market-driven demands.

Education, especially post-secondary education, must therefore train individuals who will take up various aspects of the work; otherwise the workforce will not be employable. The workforce should also be very competitive, given the demands and pressures of the marketplace. A properly trained workforce ensures that corporations and organisations become more competitive and better performing, and can better position themselves in the marketplace. In this sense, Lundvall and Johnson (1994) have argued that if knowledge is the most important resource in modern economy, then learning is its most important process. Workers—and therefore students—must be equipped with proper theory, facts, models and evidence. They must also learn and practise various skills, including effective and collaborative communication, negotiation, critical thinking, independent learning, leadership, coordination and delegation, teamwork, decision-making, problem-solving, conflict resolution, risk and crisis management, and creative innovation. Finally, they must learn to transfer these skills across various contexts, as they are likely to move from one work position to the next or from one area of specialisation to another.

The role of knowledge in relation to economic goals is well established, including in nursing. Yet it becomes obvious that concepts such as *knowledge economy, knowledge society* and *knowledge worker* teeter on the boundary between knowing and not knowing. Looking at the relationship between ignorance and economy is a different exercise if one seeks a more sophisticated understanding that moves beyond conceptualisations of ignorance-as-absence-of-knowledge. At first glance, one could simply consider ignorance itself as a tradable commodity. To be sure, ignorance can be a source of profit, inasmuch as goods and services can be developed so as to counter or manage ignorance. Numerous books, devices and experts exist because they help individuals manage things about which they are not knowledgeable, but purportedly should be. Ignorance can also be an economic driver in the form of intellectual property rights and the strategic management of trade secrets. In these cases, limiting or completely restricting other individuals' access to particular information is a common mechanism to ensure the viable profitability of certain entities (products, ideas, inventions, patents, etc.).

One can also explore the way ignorance can be tied to the preservation of economic interests in the context of contested socioeconomic practices. This is particularly evident, for instance, in the way exploitative features of capitalistic modes of production and distribution are routinely obscured in mainstream politics (understood here in the administrative–judicial sense). Ignorance can therefore be strategically sustained through the denial of class conflict, or the cloaking of indigence, violence and modern practices of slavery, leading to the obstruction of information that could otherwise endanger the unhindered operations of capitalist institutions and technologies. The plight of factory or farm workers worldwide, for example, regularly comes to light when new evidence surfaces exposing the abuse and unsafe work practices they endure (see e.g. Burke 2013; Bilton 2014; Haaretz 2015), spurring a wide array of analyses of the social, economic, historical and political repercussions of labour practices grounded in capitalism. Ignorance of the predicament of these workers is made all the easier if retailers conceal the sources of the goods they sell, and if consumers rationalise the need for these goods as an important aspect of their own sociocultural identity. This is well captured in Paharia's analysis, evocatively titled 'Sweatshop labor is wrong unless the shoes are cute', which empirically examines the way consumers use moral reasoning to justify unethical labour (and consumer) practices and to mediate their relationship with, and loyalty to, companies whose profits are derived from sweatshop activity (Paharia et al. 2013; see also Ehrich and Irwin 2005). It also illustrates the way knowledge acquisition about the specificities and inequities of workers' rights in remote territories do not automatically translate into a particular course of action, such as foregoing certain products or manufacturers because of contested labour practices. Consumption therefore rests on awareness about particular products (through advertisements), but also on the careful avoidance of knowledge that may engender moral disquiet and compromise. 'Wilful ignorance' works to construct and maintain the unfortunate labourer as an abstract entity. It also helps 'avoid the emotional and cognitive cost of incorporating knowledge of potentially unfavourable unethical attributes in [one's] decision' (Paharia et al. 2013: 82), thereby securing a complacent, and therefore compliant, client base.

The study of the relationship between ignorance and the economy can be pushed further. For example, we are just beginning to hear about the notion of *ignorance mobilisation*, namely through the work of Joanne Gaudet (2013; Gaudet et al. 2012), who advocates for a more positive view of ignorance. Before her, Joanne Roberts put forth the term *ignorance economy*, sceptically considering what she identifies as an overly optimistic view of knowledge as the main driver of capitalist economies. More specifically, Roberts demonstrates that what is commonly conceptualised as the 'knowledge economy' in fact rests and depends on 'the production, distribution, and consumption of ignorance' (Roberts and Armitage 2008: 345) as well as 'the speedy obsolescence of knowledge and thus… the expansion of ignorance' (346). Among many examples, she describes how, in advanced economies, individuals are less and less able, or required, to acquire or secure the knowledge needed to live their lives. As a result, they are increasingly dependent on others (government agencies, corporations) to collect, store and use knowledge to provide basic necessities (food, water, housing) and other products that are generally considered to be essential (cars, clocks, computers, communication devices, loans). The increase in specialisation that is required in advanced economies thus goes hand-in-hand with a parallel increase in ignorance about the production and operation of common goods (Roberts and Armitage 2008). Such ignorance therefore results in the requirement for, and increased dependence on, additional services and supports by corporations which control the knowledge about their products—and, incidentally, the quality and the longevity of those products. Ignorance, then, is tightly linked to matters of consumption. And, much like knowledge, it carries its own market value.

Ungar (2008) echoes the notion that ignorance is an inevitable consequence of the knowledge economy. He uses the expression 'knowledge–ignorance paradox' to highlight the dynamic and tumultuous relationship between the two concepts. This paradox illustrates how ignorance always increases because it constitutes a by-product of social pressures for more and more knowledge. Ungar argues that knowledge is no longer an appropriate point of departure for sociological explanations of particular phenomena; rather, ignorance must be set as the starting point. He goes so far as to say that knowledge, in fact, is the exception: in light of increased specialisation in all areas of life, knowledge, not ignorance, is the object, the anomaly requiring attention and explanation (Ungar 2008). Knowledge-generation structures are therefore 'naturally' geared towards the production of both knowledge and ignorance that can assist in the creation of new goods dedicated to marketisation. The skewing of knowledge development becomes obvious, first because it promotes certain questions over others (e.g. those that can lead to new technologies versus those seeking to understand particular phenomena; see e.g. Radder 2010); and second because it often reduces these to 'micro-questions' and therefore narrow fields of inquiry reflecting the uniqueness and exclusivity that is the trademark of specialisation.

The existence of an economy of ignorance forces us to pry open the multi-faceted mechanisms underpinning current distributions of knowledge and ignorance, and the discursive strategies that normalise and legitimise such distributions, even in the face of glaring abuse. It therefore brings us to consider the intricate inclusion and exclusion dynamics brought on by these distributions and their subject-forming power.

The morality of ignorance

It is clear that, in examining the concept of ignorance, one must devote some time and attention to its relationship with morality. In current literature, references abound to ignorance and knowledge as being grounded in morality. The moral dimension of ignorance can be examined in a number of ways. In this section both positive and negative renditions of ignorance, as discussed in various disciplines, are discussed. Discourses about ignorance and morality are principally grounded in political science, epistemology and sociology. Authors who relate these discussions to the domain of health and healthcare are few. We have found only one nursing text (published as a chapter in a book grounded in medical sciences and information services) that explicitly deals with ignorance as a moral problem for patient care (Faulkner 1985).

The negative connotations that often accompany traditional discussions about ignorance generally work to cast ignorance as a sign of failure, be it social, political or ethical. Perhaps one of the earliest conceptions of this type of ignorance is evident in the way Socrates addressed Alcibiades, whom he castigated as being ignorant, but also as being ignorant of his ignorance. Ignorance, for Socrates, was evil and shameful, and knowledge, a supreme virtue, was its only remedy (De Koninck 2000). Socrates advocated for knowledge that was gained through a dialectal method whereby one must answer a series of questions that bring one to a critique of one's beliefs in light of particular moral concepts, such as justice and truth. Such questioning therefore leads to a sincere examination of one's moral disposition and worth.

Today, such a view remains entrenched, albeit in different arrangements. Ignorance is known to exist, but it is deemed unremarkable overall, an avoidable component of modern societies that remain dedicated to improving the process of learning more about themselves and the world in which they live. Being knowledgeable has become an important goal, whether this is achieved through formal education, practical experience, institutionalised scientific ventures, or personal endeavours focused on self-discovery and awareness. There remains a dominant view that knowledge constitutes the main stimulus of one's moral compass. What is defined as knowledge, however, may vary from one author to the next. Some, such as Ungar, have a broad view of what kinds of knowledge individuals should be imbued with in order to function appropriately in society. For example, he points out that, in the knowledge economy, despite substantial advances in improving the lives of most people, 'cascading increases in knowledge are accompanied by a persistent undertow of ignorance' (2008: 301). He identifies 'functional knowledge deficits' as a troubling social issue, proposing a number of examples of such deficits, ranging from economics illiteracy to historical ignorance, to ignoring the workings of national and local politics or basic physiological processes, to being unable to make simple calculations or understand the concept of probability. Such knowledge is generally thought to be necessary for one's responsible—and moral—engagement in effective citizenship. A good citizen is knowledgeable and pragmatic, inasmuch as she uses available knowledge to achieve something beneficial and useful in society; for example, a 'worthwhile' career or the maintenance of optimal health. The moral dimension of combating ignorance becomes evident when matters of knowledge production and utilisation are embedded within specifically practical aims.

Other authors contend that what is needed is individuals' reconnection with fundamentals that help uphold their basic humanity and relationship with the world around them. De Koninck (2000) proposes that culture, philosophy and art are needed, and he disputes the capacity of science to cure concrete, everyday social ills such as poverty, alienation and violence. Furthermore, in his view, science alone cannot restore basic values such as solidarity, justice, understanding, acceptance and friendship. Modern culture rests on the persistent but growing equation of abstractions (numbers, symbols, figures) and illusions (appearances, deceptions, fantasies) with reality. De Koninck does not simply chastise contemporary (Western) popular culture, bent on celebrating particular kinds of accomplishments (wealth and stardom in particular). To him, the reduction of the complexity of life to mathematical calculations and modelling undermines one's ability to capture complexity, breeding ignorance through fractional and ultimately biased claims. Citing French philosopher Gabriel Marcel, he cautions against the capacity of such 'spirit of abstraction' to sever some aspects of life (e.g. humans) from others (e.g. nature), to isolate and decontextualise them in such a way as to render them meaningless and inconsequential. For De Koninck (2000), ignorance is an inevitable and potentially deadly product of rationalisation, reduction and abstraction: it can breed boredom, narcissism, cruelty and even war. He puts forth philosophy, ethics and arts as a powerful antidote to ongoing, yet often subtle, violations of human dignity.

Henry Giroux (2014) is similarly concerned with contemporary moral conditions. In his view, 'massive inculcation of ignorance' is not only real, it is planned, calculated, systematised, rationalised and operationalised, in the form of pseudo-news, pedagogical enterprises disguised as curriculum reforms, and intelligence gathering and management parading as national security imperatives. Giroux uses the term *amnesia* to describe the extent of contemporary manufactured misinformation and historical and political forgetting, whose danger resides in how accountability, critical thought and moral positioning are rendered void. Despite this, these processes are exceedingly powerful, producing outcasts who sink into oblivion because of their inability (interpreted as their unwillingness) to partake in consumerist citizenship. For Giroux, ignorance is a cultural by-product of market imperatives and neoliberal policies, and a catalyst for violence, oppression and war—war in the obvious sense, such as that waged on the Iraqi people on the basis of spurious facts. In a more subtle, perverted form it is war waged through cuts in public services and social programmes on low-income individuals, women, immigrants and youth—especially youth of colour, as disturbingly captured in the 'school-to-prison pipeline' metaphor (Giroux 2014: 55).

Ignorance is often cast as an obscuring force giving rise to such ideologies as racism and sexism, or to censorship, exclusion and oppression. In sociological analyses of oppressive ways of thinking, speaking and acting, parallels between ignorance and intolerance are proposed to explain the harmful effects of ignorance on particular individuals or groups. As Sullivan and Tuana point out,

> Sometimes what we do not know is not a mere gap in knowledge, the accidental result of an epistemological oversight. Especially in the case of racial oppression, a lack of knowledge or an unlearning of something previously known often is actively produced for purposes of domination and exploitation.
>
> (Sullivan and Tuana 2007: 1)

Reiterating Sullivan and Tuana, Hoagland (2007) takes care to note that such epistemologies and practices of ignorance can be formally sanctioned, codified, and provided with constitutional immunity through legal practices of ignorance portrayed as ethical and for the benefit and safety of the public. Hoagland argues that individuals located in dominant cultures (mostly Caucasian and wealthy) are actively involved in constructing and enacting epistemologies of ignorance. They sustain and defend such epistemologies through an ethics of ignorance that rests on the denial of relationality. This is in keeping with Paharia and colleagues' (2013) contention, referred to earlier. Hoagland's argument posits that epistemologies that rest on and sustain the notion of the free autonomous subject work to conceal the way subjectivities are shaped through the discursive elimination of oppressive relational mechanisms.

Knowledge, as such, is largely understood as inherently righteous; and ignorance, as lack of knowledge, as potentially leading to dire consequences. Ignorance (whatever form it may take) is largely made responsible for the enduring and devastating effects of poor health, sexual and racial discrimination, religious wars and poverty. A more sophisticated analysis leads us to consider how discrimination and wars have the effects they do because they rest on the accumulation of knowledge specifically intended for cultural or physical exclusion and erasure. In most views, ignorance remains characterised as being fraught with moral judgement, often associated with futility, idiocy and overall moral failure. To this effect, Vitebsky notes that

> often, ignorance appears as something more primordial, dark, heavy and formless. Here, 'ignorance' is not simply a category of cognition, as would be required by any philosophy of knowledge (the opposite of which could simply be a state of not knowing), but is the cognitive facet of the moral term evil.
>
> (Vitebsky 1993: 100–101)

On a more pragmatic note, Moore and Tumin (1949) explore the way ignorance functions as a necessary feature of the organisation and administration of contemporary societies. They challenge the common belief that knowledge leads to social progress, and they are sceptical of the ways 'education… has been elevated in many lay and professional circles to the status of panacea for all of man's ills' (787). They argue that ignorance is critical to effective social arrangements and dynamics, such as the codification of interactions between a specialist and a client seeking that specialist's expertise. Power differentials between the two are reflective of the division of labour (Moore and Tumin 1949), but they also provide a script for exchanges between them, thereby rendering these interactions predictable to some extent. These authors also explore the role of ignorance in the management of trade secrets or the maintenance of security if strategic knowledge is withheld from an enemy. Through the various scenarios they explore, it is clear that ignorance can be interpreted as a compulsory feature of organised social life that can result in either positive or negative outcomes, but that nonetheless provides a stabilising force throughout community and organisational networks. Ignorance can trigger creativity, maintain power differentials, provide a competitive edge, and enforce social stereotypes, leading Moore and Tumin to conclude that its status as exclusively disruptive, inhibiting or morally void is unwarranted.

John Rawls (1971) proposes a different reading of the ethical value of ignorance. In examining the way individuals choose particular courses of action, he has determined that ignorance removes those filters and reflexes that lead individuals to make self-interested decisions. Rawls uses the expression 'veil of ignorance' to describe a thought experiment in which individuals cannot know or predict their status (gender, age, race, aptitudes, etc.) in a fictional society in which they are asked to distribute such things as rights and wealth. When unable to determine how they, themselves, would fare in such a society, they are more likely to make fair decisions, as these would inevitably affect them when their position was revealed. The maintenance of ignorance therefore prevents individuals from making decisions aimed at preserving self-interest, and is constitutive of Rawls' theory of justice. Under such conditions, ignorance acts as a guardian, or a guarantor of moral thought and conduct in the writing of a new social contract. Rawls' writings appear in several nursing texts on ethics (see e.g. Basford and Slevin 2003; Benjamin and Curtis 2010; Sorrell Dinkins 2011; Ellis 2014); however, Rawls' deliberate focus on ignorance to convey a human disposition toward moral reasoning is overlooked. What remains instead is an interpretation of justice as a product of empathy and critical reflection, rather than an ideal reached through the productive properties of ignorance (see e.g. Sorrell Dinkins 2011).

We have found only one nursing text that specifically emphasises, albeit very briefly, the central and positive role of ignorance in achieving social justice (Masters 2014). For many nurse writers, especially those theorising the ethical foundations of nursing practice, it is clear that ignorance is neither a matter of epistemology nor a concept worthy of exploration. In the prevailing context of knowledge production, collection, distribution and translation, honouring the mysterious entity that is the patient and her knowledge can be construed as an act of resistance. This is so because it promotes a form of knowledge that is far more difficult to capture and explain, a move that stands in stark contrast to the calls for hard facts and strong evidence that suffuse health services management and policy work. A commitment to less codified forms of knowledge acknowledges and accepts the many realms of uncertainty—and ignorance—that lie in its wake, something that has been emphasised in much of feminist scholarship (Townley 2011) and described as an integral part of epistemic justice (Code 1991, 2008a). It fundamentally disrupts the logics of the politics of truth (in a Foucauldian sense) that govern healthcare organisations, scientific research and, more generally, current knowledge systems that structure societies. It escapes from the accepted modes of intelligibility and therefore from the subjectifying, normative and often alienating effects of technical rational forms of knowledge.

Implications of ignorance studies for nursing

Working with geographical concepts is uncommon in nursing; nursing history has been much more active in its provision of accounts and stories of nursing. Many histories address nursing through its noteworthy practitioners (such as Florence Nightingale and other nursing icons; Nelson and Rafferty 2010), and events that nurses were involved in, such as various wars, outbreaks of disease or disasters (D'Antonio 2006; Nelson 2009). There are acknowledged difficulties in writing nursing into history due to deficits in records about what nurses do in clinical settings—and we outline that lack within this book. There are growing calls to record nurses' work in practice settings (D'Antonio 2006), and to outline how knowledge was developed and influenced in genealogies of nursing knowledge (Nelson 2012)—all of which interact with what nurses did not know and how that related to calls to discover nurses' work in healthcare. We also consider how nursing uses ignorance to hide issues in Chapter 4 of this book, in the discussion of dangerous ideas. As with history, the issue is with using geographical concepts such as space, place (Carolan et al. 2006), and non-place or cyberspace (Andrews and Kitchin 2005). As with histories, a focus on places of care, and spaces where nursing happens, takes precedence, with little focus on what is not known when we use a geographical lens. Clearly, spatial aspects of care abound where nurses practise outside 'usual' settings such as hospitals, but there are few analyses that question what is known/not known when addressing the particularities of place (see Parker 2004) as this intersects with uncertainties and ambiguities (Latimer 1999).

Nursing is comfortable with enabling moral agency through the concept of 'unknowing' proposed by Munhall (1993), and reiterated by several authors in Locsin and Purnell (2009). In this view, unknowingness about the other's life equals 'openness' (Munhall 1993: 125). Unknowing is a conscious process, a form of wilful ignorance that allows a care provider to suspend one's self and accompanying beliefs, theories, values and expertise, in order to make way for the expression of a patient's self and agency. In order to do this, the care practitioner must have proper insights into what, precisely, must be 'bracketed out'. Nurses must thus reflect on their self in order to clarify their own paradigm, belief system and principles. Only then, according to Locsin and Purnell (2009) and their collaborators, can the full complexity of patients can be discerned. Through unknowing, nurses can ensure that patients, as experts of their own realities, are not 'hijacked' by care processes that may rob them of their humanity and autonomy.

Binding nursing knowledge and practice to (non)knowledge of the patient is both a risky and powerful endeavour. It is risky in the sense that such patient knowledge is unstable, shifting, unspecialised, perhaps inexplicable, and often unrecorded in traditional modes of knowledge transmission such as textbooks or scientific journals. It is subjective, uncodified and nearly impossible to quantify. Therefore, despite its value for those who uphold the aesthetic dimension of healthcare, it does not rank very highly in prevailing 'hierarchies of evidence'. After all, David Sackett, considered to be one of the founders of the evidence-based movement, did rule that 'Art kills' (Zuger 1997). Taking the position of (non)knowledge simultaneously elicits strong moral value and significance. It provides a compelling defence for a particular course of action that is at odds with prevailing 'best practice'. It places the patient squarely at the centre of care interventions and clinical objectives. It also suggests that nurses, despite the bureaucratic and technocratic turn of contemporary healthcare organisations, attempt to stay true to care ideals.

While recognising that this chapter crosses an extensive terrain of work on ignorance from different perspectives, we have attempted to provide a view of ignorance not only as a motivating force, but also as mediating how the world is thought of—a way of thinking about knowledge and its shadow. We have chosen to explore its place in historical, spatial, moral and economic dimensions, where the concept is put to work to explore social and other relations. We now turn to more in-depth explorations of ignorance in nursing and healthcare, beginning with a troublesome aspect of contemporary healthcare: uncertainty.

3 Ignorance

Knowledge interrupted

Writing a book on ignorance begins from the premise that ignorance is, indeed, recognisable as such by those who are ignorant or who ignore, and by those who bear witness to it (Code 2014). Proctor (2008: 2) argues that '[i]gnorance has many interesting surrogates and overlaps in myriad ways with—as it is generated by—*secrecy, stupidity, apathy, censorship, disinformation, faith* and *forgetfulness*, all of which are science-twitched' (emphasis in original). To Proctor's list, we add uncertainty, confidentiality, deceit and discretion. We agree with him that the concept of ignorance as it currently is considered and perceived in current academic and lay discourses provides little ground to its analysis and the analysis of its effects. If ignorance constitutes a state in which 'not all can be known', then we need to be able to broaden our approach in such a way as to include other contemporary terminologies and understandings that convey states of non-knowledge.

We have therefore elected to examine such concepts as uncertainty, denial and deceit in our exploration of the workings of ignorance in nursing and healthcare. All of these practices or states of mind share a common assumption: that valuable, desirable or necessary knowledge is either required but not available, or available but not to be circulated, thereby inducing a state of non-knowledge in others. In other words, all of these terms imply an inter-ruption in the flow of knowledge. They are powerful to the extent that, much like knowledge, each steers possible courses of action in a particular direction. Nursing-as-boundary-work is clearly articulated in various ways through nursing researchers' and scholars' efforts in delineating the boundaries and the legitimacy of nursing science and knowledge, but also in exploring the ways in which these play out in clinical, educational and administrative spaces.

Uncertainty and its capacity to saturate everyday life

In healthcare in general, and nursing in particular, uncertainty has generated copious scholarship addressing it as a problem. Much of the literature we reviewed discusses it as a 'fact of life' in physical and emotional care situations, an unavoidable condition that practitioners and patients must grapple with when making decisions (see e.g. Mishel 1981; Curley et al. 1984; Baumann et al.

1991; Penrod 2001, 2007; Thompson and Dowding 2001; Benner et al. 2009; Locsin and Purnell 2009; Vaismoradi et al. 2010; Waska 2011). Smith (1992: 134) notes that 'the complexity of healthcare may make it intrinsically unpredictable: we may never be able to know what we would like to know'. Uncertainty is described as both an individual and a collective response in the face of indeterminate events, such as fluctuating biological processes (e.g. pathogenic, hemodynamic) or organisational phenomena (e.g. restructuring). With uncertainty comes varying states of confidence and sense of control over a given situation and various, perhaps conflicting, cognitive and emotional interpretations of probable and desirable outcomes (Penrod 2007). Current analyses tend to focus on uncertainty as a subjective experience, linked to perceptions of various environmental cues. In this literature, uncertainty is largely depicted as an awkward sensation, one that can spur actions that will lead to positive outcomes, including the alleviation of discomfort and anxiety associated with a (perceived) lack of knowledge and control. Thus it is clear that we, as individuals, patients, practitioners, administrators and decision-makers, recognise the pervasiveness of uncertainty in our daily lives. Bourgeault (1999), however, questions whether we truly come to grips with it.

It is unsurprising, then, that much contemporary research and policy development aims precisely at either eliminating uncertainty as it arises in clinical or organisational situations, or carefully managing it so as to limit potential negative outcomes. Some authors have suggested that uncertainty is focused on the present (Penrod 2001, 2007; Vaismoradi et al. 2010); that is, practitioners struggle with uncertainty in the here and now, at the very moment when a course of action is required, and when they cannot confidently choose a particular one. This temporal distinction is important; however, along with Beck (1992) and Giddens (1991, 1999), we argue that, because of its close relationship with risk assessment and management, uncertainty is also future-oriented. This view allows us to capture how various (non)knowledges, assumptions and hopes bring an uncertain future into the modifiable present—modifiable through a logic of rationalisation and utility maximisation so as to decrease the likelihood of unfortunate events (Giddens 1991; Buchak 2013). However, one cannot fully appreciate the impact of uncertainty without contrasting its meaning in relation to its location in a risk-averse society.

In contemporary culture, especially Western culture, risk management is both a local and a global matter, both an individual and a collective affair, something that, in today's 'global risk landscape' (Beck and Holzer 2007: 5), requires an adequate response. No matter which conceptualisation of risk is privileged, whether grounded in social constructionism or realism, it is clear that risk and its administration are chief concerns for the modern social agent, may she be a lay individual, healthcare practitioner, economist or policymaker (Beck 1992). Risks have permeated our way of thinking and behaving so deeply that one is hard pressed to explain why one does not heed the warnings against poor eating habits, does not breastfeed one's baby, walks alone at night, does not get immunised against various diseases, or does not 'take control' of one's life.

Despite their elusive, undetermined nature, risks are increasingly treated as actual fact. Disease risk is treated as if risk is the disease itself. For example, hypercholesterolemia (high levels of cholesterol in the blood), long thought to be associated with cardiovascular disease, is treated as a disease in its own right, with its own treatment (e.g. statin therapy). We are all vulnerable to developing one condition or other, from stroke to depression, from osteoporosis to cancer. And such disease continuum is exceptionally effective in blurring the lines between healthy, vulnerable and diseased states, and in conflating various subject states: non-patient, pre-patient and patient.

These various messages are powerful, for many reasons. First, they resonate with the reality and complexity of everyday life. Everyone feels concerned, because risk concerns everyone. Second, they appeal to a sense of duty and moral obligation, which spells specific modes of actions on the part of responsible citizens (Perron et al. 2005). In this instance, risk evaluation and management is consistent with the collective commitment to look out for one another. This means, however, that just as expectations regarding the care and protection of fellow citizens can travel along social channels, so too can blame (Douglas 1992). Third, these messages induce states of vulnerability requiring urgent actions that are within every person's reach, from daily walks to proper sleep, from preventive statin therapy to educational websites for anger and anxiety management. Fourth, risk management discourses appeal to reason and logic, a discursive prerequisite in order to speak to the Modern subject. What rational person would not do anything in their power to tilt the scales in their favour? Finally, they are relentless, infiltrating every aspect of our lives: magazine articles cautioning against the potentially deleterious consequences of poor diet; media reports about terror threats; salespersons advising customers to buy extended product warranty; insurance companies proposing comprehensive coverage plans; security companies promoting home alarm systems; travel agents urging vacationers to acquire health insurance; business owners installing security cameras in public areas such as stores, parking lots and fire escapes; and, more recently, therapists, life coaches and spiritual guides cautioning clients against future existential regrets, which can be prevented through self-examination, rationalisation and thoughtful action. The common thread in these instances is that ignorance and anxiety stemming from uncertainty can be abated, in an apparently linear fashion, through reason and choice. As Beck argues,

> Against the background of this growing unawareness and non-knowledge in the wake of the modernization of knowledge, the question of deciding in a context of uncertainty arises in a radical way... a society based on knowledge and risk opens up a threatening sphere of possibilities. Everything falls under an imperative of avoidance.

> (Beck 2000: 217)

Two examples can be put forth to see how ignorance generated by avoidance is at the core of risk management: sexual education, and the now defunct

'Don't Ask Don't Tell' policy of the US military. Both examples also resonate with our earlier discussion on the close relationship between ignorance and morality, and are revisited in our discussion on dangerous knowledge and taboos in Chapter 4. Houppert (1999) observes how, in many American schools, enduring ignorance about menstruation, sex, sexually transmitted diseases, pregnancy and sexual violence is a prominent feature of sex education pro- grammes (many of which must be taught by nurses) in the name of moral hygiene and proper conduct. Withholding knowledge about such issues is presented as a sure way of protecting young minds—especially girls'—against the depravity of precocious sexual explorations. Despite longstanding evidence that such strategy is counterproductive to sexual safety and wellbeing, and that comprehensive education programmes are cost-effective in the long run (Wang et al. 2000), such an approach rests on the idea that the withholding of accurate information helps protect the integrity, morality and purity of young students (Houppert 1999; Connell and Hunt 2010). The control of women's and girls' bodies, sexuality and reproductive capacity through curtailed knowledge and education is a powerful echo of Schiebinger's (2008) exploration of the lack of transfer of information about abortifacients from colonies to imperial powers. Schiebinger's analysis highlights the way such information from indigenous groups was depicted as lacking moral value, a lack that was compounded by opposition to their use set by dominant moral action regarding sexual practices and their specifically reproductive value. Reinforcement of taboos associated with sexual activity is embedded in social constructs about who is allowed to embody the sexual subject (e.g. the adult who is duly married), albeit in bounded and socially regulated ways (e.g. with only one partner of the other sex, preferably for the purposes of reproduction). Sexual norms are thus established through knowledge that prescribes and governs how, when and with whom one is authorised to engage in a sexual manner. Norms and taboos can be powerfully enforced through abstinence-only discourses promoting moral and religious ideals, and punitive actions (e.g. public shaming) towards those who violate these norms. The deployment of ignorance through the holding and avoidance of morally damaging information is therefore, above all, a strategy for the management of specific risks to morality.

Following the work of Mary Douglas, Smithson (1989: 8) argues that 'Taboos function as guardians of purity and safety through socially sanctioned rules of (ir)relevance.' They help restore order through the policing of certain kinds of knowledge, whose significance is redefined according to encoded moral imperatives as normative value. Subjects become disciplined in their manner of being, thinking and speaking, and therefore amplify the effects of ignorance as an organising framework of discourses and subjects. Moore and Tumin (1949) further point out that in any structure that deploys normative prescriptions, ignorance of deviations from the norms themselves is also to be expected, because '[a] normative system as such may suffer more from knowledge of violations than from the violations themselves' (1949: 791). This, they say, may be especially true in the case of sexual conduct, whereby knowledge of non-conforming behaviours may motivate further noncompliance, and therefore weaken the prevailing power structure. We further explore ideas around boundaries, taboos and their emotional import for ignorance in Chapter 4 of this book.

Avoidance of risks through ignorance, as something both moral and protective, has also been used as justification for the 'Don't Ask Don't Tell' policy in the US military, a policy that allowed homosexual and bisexual individuals to serve in the army so long as they did not disclose their sexual orientation and did not engage in sexual relations. Similarly, recruitment and commanding officers were barred from asking serving officers about their sexual orientation. Until the repeal of the policy in 2011, individuals were only allowed to serve under the covenant of secrecy; should their sexual orientation be known, they were discharged from military service. The maintenance of ignorance in this case was deemed necessary because

> The presence in the armed forces of persons who demonstrate a propensity or intent to engage in homosexual acts would create an unacceptable risk to the high standards of morale, good order and discipline, and unit cohesion that are the essence of military capability.
>
> (US Government 1993: 127).

In the same vein, ignorance about a serving officer's sexual orientation was purported to be protective inasmuch as officers could not be discriminated against. In both this scenario and that of sexual education, it is noteworthy that the supposed protective feature of ignorance through avoidance is said to benefit young girls and homosexuals in particular, two groups whose sexuality is routinely depicted as socially and morally dangerous and as needing to be carefully reined in.

Science versus uncertainty—small comfort

Contemporary discourses about risk management imply that through careful, rational weighting of information, one can make appropriate choices. Choice refers to a decision based on purportedly calculable probabilities, in a world of increasing social, political and technological complexity and change (Lupton 1999). And while science, technological advances and industrialisation generate their contemporary brand of uncertainty, one may find comfort in the Modern way of thinking that science can—will—also provide answers and solutions (Giddens 1991; Beck 1995). Modern living, then, resembles a broad exercise in problem-solving through information gathering, decision-making, and taking responsibility for these decisions (Lupton 1999).

In clinical settings such calculation resonates in particular ways, inasmuch as 'appropriate decisions', such as forming diagnosis A or B, or following course of treatment 1 or 2, bear important consequences in the short and long term for patients and practitioners alike. In order to help care recipients and health professionals navigate this complex process, various tools have been proposed, from clinical guidelines to decision aids. Despite their highly author-itative nature, such tools are only imperfect or provisional, to the extent that the required evidence to develop them may be absent, or may be deemed incon-clusive or of poor quality (French 2002; Knaapen 2013). As numerous studies dealing with multiple issues are disseminated every day, 'old' evidence must be reappraised, compared, weighed against new findings, and ultimately updated or discarded. Evidentiary knowledge is impermanent, and continuously subjected to the development of new knowledge, new insights and new assessment tools (Roberts and Armitage 2008; Jensen 2014). In Firestein's words,

> No datum is safe from the next generation of scientists with the next generation of tools. The known is never safe; it is never quite sufficient... a definitive prediction is more likely to be wrong than a vague one that allows several possible outcomes.
>
> (Firestein 2012: 21)

Individual behaviours and organisational practices aimed at managing uncer-tainty and risk may well rest on poor scientific evidence, but are often perceived as still better than 'doing nothing'. Science is meant to produce facts, proof, certainty, confirmation and assurance. It may lead to more questions, but it is expected first and foremost to yield answers. Scientific production is thought to eliminate uncertainties (Code 2013) and can therefore lead to the devising of a particular course of action in the shape of a standardised guideline, institutional protocol or treatment algorithm.

Scientific knowledge attempts to secure expanding realms of knowledge and push back the figurative frontiers where knowledge and ignorance meet. As Ungar (2008: 317) points out, 'in so far as the dominant public discourse recognizes uncertainties and ignorance in scientific knowledge, these are seen as resolvable over time rather than endemic and irreducible'. As a dominant discourse and powerful organiser of social, economic and political life, science can make claims to establish its dominance, identify its shortcomings and, remarkably, posit itself as the solution to its own limits. The problems of such circular logic have been captured by Dreyfus and Rabinow, who sceptically note that 'We are promised normalization and happiness through science and law. When they fail, this only justifies the need for more of the same' (1982: 196).

Bourgeault (1999) highlights how the current dominance of technical rationality in Modern societies has given precedence to the questions of *how* and *how much*, but that other important questions, such as *what, why* and *whom*, which explicitly work to underscore the fundamental humanness of the world we live in, remain largely unexplored. This is also true in current health services research and governance, where there has been a definite departure from social, ethical and philosophical questions, toward investigation focused on health service efficiency, efficacy, sustainability, technological transforma-tion, and the translation of findings into marketable innovations (Rose 2007). Ethical and philosophical questions, aside from not being particularly profitable, do not lend themselves very well to a quest for certitude. In Canada, over the past decade, research on various phenomena—such as chronic poverty, environmental crises, drug safety, women's issues, and the realities of minority groups—has been directly and indirectly excluded from the federal research agenda, with the cancelling or rededication of funds formerly devoted to these issues (see e.g. Sheikh 2011; Singh 2014). Efforts to silence knowledge development in some key areas of human life, or more precisely, such maintenance of ignorance in specific areas, becomes all the more justified when it is discursively constructed as protecting or promoting 'good science' as opposed to 'pseudo-science'. Good science is apparently tied to industry interests and control (Radder 2010).

Despite, or because of, such a contested context of science production, uncertainty remains a significant aspect of health and health work. In nursing, it constitutes an important focus of current scholarship, especially that grounded in evidence-based practice, decision-making and administration. Uncertainty, as a form of ignorance, is depicted as a clinical problem because it is said to be responsible for significant practice variations, which then lead to inconsistent and suboptimal clinical outcomes. French (2002), for example, argues that practitioner uncertainty, which she defines as the state in which a health practitioner is unsure about the best course of action, results in uneven clinical decision-making. She goes on to say that one of the assumptions about evidence-based healthcare, which aims to provide healthcare providers with 'best evidence', is that it will lead to fewer variations and better results. Here uncertainty, especially practitioner uncertainty, is considered a significant (clinical) problem with serious implications regarding quality patient care.

Uncertainty may arise in a number of ways. Nurses and other health professionals work 'in an environment that is already riddled with uncertainty about professional identity, roles and the management of risk' (French 2002: 251). They must also manage unforeseen clinical events on a daily basis, as well as changes to their workplace, such as the implementation of new policies, changes in staff ratios, or even patient arrival rate (we return to this situation in Chapter 6). New graduates experience heightened uncertainty as they attempt to navigate what has been termed the 'theory–practice gap' (Saltzberg 2002)—the mismatch between what they learned during their formative years and what they face as professionals (Rafferty et al. 1996). It is clear from current nursing literature that nurses should follow up on feelings of uncertainty and seek to acquire the necessary information to act appropriately, and that doing otherwise puts patients at risk. This is consistent with longstanding calls in nursing to engage in introspection and reflective practice, which allows nurses to privately and autonomously identify knowledge gaps and learning needs. As seen earlier, decision aids and clinical guidelines are said to support nurses in their efforts to be more knowledgeable professionals by alleviating knowledge-related uncertainties.

What is often missing from such analyses is the way knowledge (and lack thereof) constitute nurses as particular subjects—knowledge users—tied to particular practice scenarios, where knowledge management is key in safe and effective patient care. As Kerwin (1993) argues, while people are generally in agreement regarding the limits of science and the accompanying vastness of ignorance, they are far less tolerant of health practitioner ambivalence and fallibility, arguing that it is their responsibility to keep up to date with relevant research in order to properly address individuals' physical and emotional ailments and, at times, their uncertain futures. Such perception focuses on ignorance and uncertainty as individual traits to be overcome—mainly through the use of 'authorised' knowledge in the form of best practice guidelines and decision models (Baumann et al. 1991; Thompson and Dowding 2001; French 2002; Vaismoradi et al. 2010). In contemporary healthcare organisations, such tools remain decisively grounded in positivist epistemology. This is in keeping with the received view that such science can best provide answers to most, if not all, problems. As such, descriptive and normative positions regarding proper clinical practice remain; and despite the fact that clinical judgement and other 'unscientific' sources of knowledge are said to play an important role in practice, discourses of research and guideline development continue routinely to highlight the problems and dangers of practices that are not evidence-based and not based on a hierarchy of specific kinds of evidence.

In nursing, few authors have examined the power/knowledge relationships that underpin these discourses, and the ensuing subordination of nurses to knowledge-seeking behaviours. Several authors have taken issue with the epistemological and political aspects of the rational–technical alignment of evidence-based medicine and its hopeful claim to provide practitioners with sound, unbiased and rigorous evidence (Every-Palmer and Howick 2014; for an extensive review see Miles et al. 2008). However, few have explicitly examined this from the perspective of ignorance as it plays out in prevailing discourses about what constitutes 'knowing' and 'not knowing'—a focus in Chapter 6 of this book, where relations between research practice, knowledge use and audit are examined from the perspective of ignorance. Rational solutions continue to dominate current conceptualisations of quality practice, yet more and more scholars and practitioners argue that personal, 'feeling' knowledge, in the form of experiences or intuition, remains paramount to proper decision-making and risk management, so as to not leave us 'too coldly rational' (Slovic et al. 2004: 320). Unsurprisingly, however, such orientations have been refuted—with abundant references to science—as unreliable (Grove et al. 2000).

Ignorance in the messiness of social transactions

In the situation of how the social is affected by uncertainty, decisions about what knowledge counts as valid, or not, fall under the auspices of epistemology, philosophy and sociology, rather than medical science. However, as Hulme (2007) astutely observes, 'debates about… wider social values… masquerade as disputes about scientific truth and error'. Such debates touch on issues that run deeper than proper methodology; they turn on how we circumscribe human nature, intellect and values, and how these shape efforts to capture the world as we (think we) know it. Theoretical tools grounded in a technical rational paradigm may not prove very useful in real-world clinical scenarios because of the messiness of human experiences. Such experiences, much like those faced by nurses on a daily basis, are value-laden, convoluted and ramifying; they do not necessarily spell a scientifically backed solution; and a nurse's ability to handle such situations may well rest on large amounts of ignorance. As Schön argues:

> We can readily understand, therefore, not only why uncertainty, uniqueness, instability, and value conflict are so troublesome to the Positivist epistemology of practice, but also why practitioners bound by this epistemology find themselves caught in a dilemma... In the varied topography of professional practice, there is a high, hard ground where practitioners can make effective use of research-based theory and technique, and there is a swampy lowland where situations are confusing 'messes' incapable of technical solution. The difficulty is that the problems of the high ground are often relatively unimportant to clients or larger society, while in the swamp are the problems of greatest human concern.
>
> (Schön 1988: 67)

In managing human, 'messy' clinical situations, nurses navigate, manage and mediate simultaneously multiple forms of knowledge. They are, indeed, knowledge workers, but not in the sense that management experts conceptualise it—not in the sense of participating in the production and consumption of knowledge such as clinical data or practice guidelines. In our view, nurses' 'knowledge work' is less formalised, less circumscribed by professional standards, institutional requirements or scientific authority, less rational-technical; it is more fluid, visceral, and usually an improvised response to what they see before them. And most, if not all, of their 'knowledge work' rests on the management of their or others' non-knowing.

Firstly, nursing work revolves heavily around information regarding patients' health state. This is captured, for example, in the way the nursing process is said to begin with robust data collection, including subjective information (e.g. past medical history, current symptoms, health habits) that patients may not wish to disclose. Without such knowledge, the clinical process embodied in the therapeutic encounter comes to a halt. The stakes involved are all too evident when the flow of clinical work is disturbed or interrupted because a patient fails to answer questions and provide the knowledge needed to pursue clinical actions. Nurses are trained to communicate effectively with patients in order to establish a climate of trust conducive to disclosure. Such aspects are particularly salient in contexts where patients are deemed to pose a risk to their own or others' safety. Discomfort and frustration are common because patients' silence falls outside the ritualistic nature of clinical interviews and the norms and expectations that regulate them. Such behaviour clearly disrupts the smooth running of clinical practice and the health setting itself, which rests on the steady and predictable circulation of knowledge to achieve both its pastoral and disciplinary goals (Perron et al. 2005).

Secondly, nurses and other health practitioners must uphold strict rules regarding patient confidentiality and privacy laws, which, in essence, work to maintain a form of secrecy over privileged matters. As ruled by the Supreme Court of Canada in Halls v. Mitchell (1928: 136), and which extends to all healthcare practitioners,

> Nobody would dispute that a secret so acquired is the secret of the patient, and, normally, is under his control, and not under that of the doctor. *Prima facie*, the patient has the right to require that the secret shall not be divulged; and that right is absolute, unless there is some paramount reason which overrides it.

Bok (1989) adds that at the centre of confidentiality claims lie claims to control of one's personal domain. This is particularly consistent with the claim to self-government inherent in the Western ideal of the autonomous subject. Consequently, patient confidentiality induces states of ignorance inasmuch as it places ethical and legal restrictions on the sharing of knowledge outside patient care or legal proceedings. Nurses make daily calls about the appropriateness of sharing particular information with other clinicians, family members, public health authorities, child welfare officials or the police, with deep consequences for patients. And while confidentiality is often heralded as protective of patients' rights and wellbeing, Bok cautions that such a view is naïve at best because of the fine line between confidentiality and deception:

> The sick, the poor, the mentally ill, the aged, and the very young are in a paradoxical situation in this respect. While their right to confidentiality is often breached and their most intimate problems bandied about, the poor care they may receive is just as often covered up under the same name of confidentiality. That is the shield held forth to prevent outsiders from finding out about negligence, overcharging, unnecessary surgery, or institutionalization. And far more than individual mistakes and misdeeds are thus covered up, for confidentiality is also the shield that professionals invoke to protect incompetent colleagues and negligence and unexpected accidents.
>
> (Bok 1983: 30)

This brings us to a third instance, whereby nurses, as well as other healthcare professionals, often find themselves in situations where patients' right to know is challenged. For example, a nurse may receive instructions from a physician not to disclose or discuss a diagnosis or particular events (e.g. transfer to another facility; death of a loved one) with a patient; in other situations, it is family members who wish to keep such information from the patient being cared for (Tuckett 2004; Hancock et al. 2007). Disclosing medical errors or near misses to patients has traditionally been discouraged as it was thought to undermine patients' trust in healthcare institutions—a point that was recently raised in the UK, for example, in the wake of the Francis Report, which prompted the development of guidelines on the 'duty of candour' (NMC and GMC 2014). While nurses may readily engage in such practices, chiefly in the name of the beneficence and non-maleficence principles (Tuckett 2004), it is also well known that they are often subjected to a number of censoring practices to discourage them from speaking out about organisational issues with patients or the public at large, therefore enforcing a code of silence and perpetuating practices that are likely to be unethical, illegal, dangerous or violent (Ahern and McDonald 2002; Perron et al. 2004). Failure to disclose health- or treatment-related information or practice errors to patients is construed as deceptive practice.

In healthcare and beyond, deception (much like ignorance) is routinely depicted as a moral problem, especially as framed by professional practice standards. We do not wish to discuss whether requests or efforts to withhold sensitive or potentially damaging information are morally justified; this has been covered at length elsewhere (e.g. Hope 1995; Teasdale and Kent 1995; Tuckett 1998, 2004). We are more interested in the way such requirements, and one's decision to abide by or to challenge them, can have productive effects; that is, they produce 'something' of value to either an individual or an organisation, that may or may not be morally justified. It is, however, possible to conceive of deception as a course of action not exclusively grounded in maleficence.

Famed sociologist Erving Goffman (1969), for example, showed that everyday interactions are mediated by stylised performances that allow individuals to maintain certain appearances in particular social functions. In his view, discretionary and deceptive performances are a necessity of everyday life, because they help individuals strategically maintain roles, functions and interactions that are laden with social, moral and political significance. Such interactions depend on the sharing with others, and the concomitant withholding, of certain kinds of knowledge. Decisions as to whether to reveal or keep private about oneself help shape one's identity and give meaning to one's place in the world. Ignorance is therefore a key component of this fundamentally social process. Varenne (2009: 339) reiterates this point by observing that 'Sociability is moved by the ignorance that keeps revealing itself in the conduct of everyday life.' Nurses, as part of the social, enrol in these arrangements. The way they present themselves to others (for example as professional, available, understanding or busy) pre-empts all social interactions and shapes the way these unfold. There may be 'deception' in the way nurses present themselves, but this is productive in the context of exchanges that are ritualistic and bound by gender and class processes, such as those taking place within healthcare organisations. Nurses can also assist patients in the process of presentation of self. Nurses and other healthcare professionals regularly encounter patients who carefully control how they present aspects of themselves, and require caregivers to do the same.

For example, many persons prefer to conceal the fact that they have been diagnosed with socially damaging conditions such as mental health issues or HIV/AIDS, or have been interned in a drug recovery programme or a correctional facility. Both discretion and deception can be conceived of as a way of strategically managing knowledge and ignorance, managing those who can know to an extent, and cannot know to another extent. One is consciously and actively selecting the information to be shared with others, according to a subjective evaluation of uncertain risks and gains in a given interaction with a non-knower. This involves another set of relations and transactions between different kinds of knowers. 'The security of individuals may depend upon ignorance by others of personal attributes or past experiences that have no intrinsic bearing on his [*sic*] present status but which would be regarded unfavourably if known' (Moore and Tumin 1949: 790–791). Knowledge, ignorance and power are linked here too because, as Bok claims, control over knowledge provides

> a safety valve for individuals in the midst of communal life – some influence over transactions between the world of personal experience and the world shared with others. With no control over such exchanges, human beings would be unable to exercise choice about their lives… these efforts at control permeate all human contact. Those who lose all control over these relations cannot flourish in either the personal or the shared world, nor retain their sanity. If experience in the shared world becomes too overwhelming, the sense of identity suffers.
>
> (Bok 1989: 20)

Preserving others' ignorance about such facts is construed as a necessary, moral step to the preservation of one's safe and meaningful inclusion in society, where choices can be made as proper enactments of citizenship. Where negative consequences, such as retribution, stigma or marginalisation, are a very real and damaging possibility, the upholding of ignorance through non-disclosure (confidentiality, deception and discretion) constitutes a valuable strategy for negotiating risky interpersonal exchanges and preserving one's sense of self. Such types of ignorance can therefore be understood as an important, even requisite feature of complex social arrangements; and various forms of ethical reasoning can be offered as justification for their social value.

These processes, of course, can work in reverse. While they can serve patients' interests in the face of sensitive social interactions, they can also work to maintain them in disempowered states, which shields nurses and other care providers from patients challenging their care, questioning treatment or refusing interventions. Maintaining such dynamics in nurse–patient relationships falls within social expectations (which include nurses' expectations) of patients acting as passive recipients of care, which in turn ensures the smooth operations of healthcare provision (Hope 1995; Teasdale and Kent 1995). It is an exercise of power that leaves patients outside those processes where strategic judgments are made about them (Glen 1997).

Nurses may resort to various forms of non-disclosure in their day-to-day practice. In doing so, they operate as knowing agents who can evade uncertain, conflicted or damaging situations. In navigating the rules, both spoken and unspoken, surrounding uncertainty, confidentiality and deception, nurses effectively tread the line between knowledge and ignorance; they regulate transactions between individuals and the social world of healthcare; they manage the fluid boundaries between the private realm and the public domain; and in so doing they also manage patient identities and subjectivities through complex interplays between power and knowledge, as Bok highlights above. This is so because ethical principles such as confidentiality and beneficence can both activate and inhibit the gaze (in a Foucauldian sense) of the clinical apparatus to which the patient is methodically, caringly, subjected.

Conclusion

Steering through the dynamics described above is not facilitated by obtaining more knowledge. It is not exclusively the incremental or exponential increase in knowledge experienced by nurses that enables them to be active in such effects, but also the ability to harness and distribute ignorance across a wide range of actors, within a wide range of situations. In all of these examples, nurses manage closure and openness, and issues around selfhood; they uphold the primacy of the sovereign subject—sovereign because rational—and therefore they mediate relationships between citizens and the state. What the situations raised above do highlight, however, is nurses' pivotal role in mediating the flow of knowledge—risky, damaging knowledge in the eyes of physicians, administrators, patients or family members—and therefore their own position as strategic agents in the maintenance (or remediation) of non-knowing, for instance through revelation, omission, denial or deception. And whether nurses choose one course of action or another, they set in motion a set of events and a range of understandings, calculations and decisions; they mobilise ideas, interests and anxieties; and they elicit various effects by forcing the (re)distribution of power among various agents. Hence, in our view, nurses learn to 'work' knowledge in various productive ways that have multiple ramifications for all agents involved: patients, family members, administrators and so on.

Rather than referring to nurses as 'knowledge users', we prefer to refer to them as *epistemic agents* (Townley 2011), a term that better captures a form of knowledge management that is less codified, less commodified in the context of modern healthcare organisations, and more adaptable to political analyses of ignorance not confined to the realm of rational–technical thinking. Limiting discussions to restrictive and normative understandings of knowledge maintains ignorance about the salience of power, knowledge and ignorance and their interplay in professional endeavours. It maintains what Code (2014: 675) calls 'an apparently seamless epistemic imaginary'—a view, optimistic and comforting no doubt, that silences the messy transactions between epistemic agents and their world, and that rests on the belief that social transactions respond to forces that are entirely rational, entirely knowable, and entirely manageable with the proper scientific evidence, policy and leadership. We now turn to situations in healthcare work where such comforts are destabilised and emotions are acknowledged as central to the twin aspects of ignorance and knowledge.

4 Abjection, taboo and dangerous knowledge

As we have shown previously, ignorance does not occur only through what is known/unknown, but gets caught up in social relations and discussions about what can/should be known. In this chapter, our focus is on the range of ignorance(s) that underpin societal belief systems and values that nurses and other healthcare professionals hold in common with their social milieu. For this reason alone, such ignorance is based on widely held views and beliefs that prove remarkably resistant to education and clinical supervision of healthcare workers. Examples of such beliefs are taboos that are sets of beliefs or practices whose source of control is at best unknown, or at least taken for granted. Moreover, nurses' practices are often located in areas where suppressed and/ or discredited forms of knowledge exist and function as ignorance. Social taboos and associated suppressed knowledge(s) operate discursively, positioning nurses alongside groups who are excluded and marginalised because of their experiential knowledge which is deemed threatening/dangerous (e.g. Indigenous groups; people diagnosed with a mental illness or HIV/AIDS; those with differing physical or intellectual abilities).

Such experiential knowledge delimits rules regarding what can be spoken about and, therefore, what can be done or achieved clinically. Hence we outline how ignorance fostered in order to contain the abject plays a vital role as a strategy of self-preservation, enabling healthcare workers to distance themselves when faced with its unacknowledged horrors. In working with what society deems as taboo or outside the 'normal', nurses are located with what society deems as horrific—death, frightening disease conditions and disgusting bodily excreta viewed as polluting or out of place. In these cases, nurses and other health professionals are cast as abject (that is, in relation to the unaccountable, uncanny or ambiguous). While they witness these horrors, nurses work every day to cast aside atrocities such as horrific injuries, violence, suffering and agony, child abuse and other 'assaults' on their values and convictions. Distancing oneself from certain situations, while suppressing feelings of dread or repulsion, helps maintain a 'safe zone', mitigates the impact of daily assaults on the self, and safeguards health providers' ability to care for patients and also for themselves.

Collectively, the concepts we explore in this chapter traverse emotional and ethical terrains of nursing and healthcare work that are routinely discounted or considered too threatening to confront directly. Firstly, the psychoanalytic concept of abjection is suggested as a way into rarely addressed emotional reactions that spawn avoidance or stigmatisation. Abjection is a defence mechanism, a 'normal' reaction caused by behaviours or bodily matter that evoke disgust, leading us to pull away from the aversive entity. But, as we know from the fascination of some with horror movies, that which horrifies is equally capable of drawing us in; it captivates as much as it revolts. This fascination may draw one into nursing, or become a reason for leaving (Alavi 2005). Kristeva (1982) asserts that the emotion of abjection is the emotional primer on which many other emotional responses are built, and triggers other defences to avoid, disavow or substitute more civilised reactions to things that cause disgust.

Many objects that cause abject responses are related to matter that society views as taboo, as signalling the disorder of 'matter out of place' (Douglas 2002). Discussion of such matters is mediated by rules and guidance about what is improper and to be excluded according to etiquette. Healthcare workers whose work is associated with taboo objects or subjects can be included as polluted, or be excluded because they deal with such (dis)order, thus increasing opportunities for ignoring taboo topics. Indeed, we could argue that the very ideas used to discuss the emotive topics in this chapter are dangerous and destabilising. We highlight in the final sections of this chapter how such dangerous ideas and conceptualisations have created a politics of ignorance around bodies, the emotional responses to them, and the devaluing of the work that healthcare workers perform with abjected bodies. Finally, the discussion in this chapter challenges the supposed objectivity of nursing work and its associated 'professional' dispositions, leading to a more dynamic politics of knowledge/ignorance that centres nurses' roles in body work as residing in a zone of dangerous ideas. This zone acknowledges that emotions cannot be objectified, professional distance is never complete and the power of ignorance is represented by all of that remains unknown, and incomprehensible. The uncanny is one of the many dangerous ideas we attempt to ignore and sublimate in overcoming taboo, horror and sanitising our responses to the abject. Unless the abject is recognised through our embodied response, we cannot say we, as nurses, appreciate the horrors patients encounter.

Defining abjection, taboo and what is dangerous

The concepts explored in this chapter combine to address how the abject body and its correlate defence, abjection, sustain ignorance, its politics and what is, or cannot, be known in the dynamics of care in nursing and healthcare. The politics of ignorance resides in how abjection remains an unacknowledged primer for all other emotions we experience, particularly those that make sense of our embodiment (Kristeva 1982). In avoiding this emotion, its power forces nurses to contain the abject body, focusing on its boundaries and orifices, where the interior meets the exterior (e.g. the mouth, anus and sweat glands), that provides a map of the intersections of the unknown, uncanny and ambiguous across the abject body. Ignorance figures in how this emotion is displaced or disavowed (a process of denial), or sublimated (a process where horrified responses are actively transformed into more socially acceptable sense-making actions and discourses, such as turning to scientific understandings about bodily excreta, or tying nursing practice narratives to moral codes of self-sacrifice and devotion). In the containment of such anxieties and bodily problems, nurses use these defence mechanisms to make their work possible. However, the problem for nurses and other healthcare workers with the abject and abjection is that neither the processes we use to manage its anxieties, nor distancing from patients perceived as abject, resolves its problematic properties/effects. The ambiguity of abjection results from its power to horrify and its role as a defence. To complicate matters further, abjection can be understood only through the understanding and identification of knowledge considered to be dangerous or discredited by the *status quo* of healthcare politics, as well as centred in the presence of taboos and stigma for nurses and their patients.

Contact with pollution is always already accompanied by disgust (Kristeva 1982; Miller 1998); it resides outside of language, allowing only liminal positions in the in-between. Such positioning signals the need to be clean and proper as we deal with disgusting, excreted material, or with bodies considered as potentially polluting (e.g. menstruating bodies, or corpses certified as dead but not yet purified and rendered sacred by death rituals; Quested and Rudge 2001). Moreover, bodies are distinguished through hierarchies of disgust (Kristeva 1982; Miller 1998) wherein some bodies are perceived as more horrifying than others. Associated with the feminine, the abject is adjudged as governing children learning social mores and proper control of their bodies through the civilising maternal function. It is important to note that abjection does not originate from this interaction; instead it is a defence against the anxiety and *jouissance* (or pleasure) that this civilisation process causes (Kristeva 1982). Abjection is a curious mix of known and unknown. It sustains ignorance through the ways we cannot discern how the abject shapes our reactions to matter out of place (Kristeva 1982; Douglas 2002).

For the purposes of this chapter, the in-depth details that the abject and abjection play in child development will not be discussed (for more detailed analysis see Holmes et al. 2006b; Rudge and Holmes 2010). More cogent to this chapter on the unknown and abjection, it is noteworthy that relations between the body and psyche develop before language, between the structures of the psyche that govern the civilisation of the child. As Chanter (2006) highlights, in taking the concept of abjection to a more discursive position between subject and object, between known and unknown, to a space available before our subjectivities are set, before social structures take over our identification, we are able to conceive of what is abject, yet jettisoned, disavowed when we fail to acknowledge the position and discourse that abjection affords and produces. These are dangerous ideas, where bodies and their products are central to the discussion, where the power of patriarchy is confronted, where the maternal function is apprehended as powerful despite all that marginalises motherhood and children as well as marginalised men. Moreover, refusing the abject is only ever partial, its power lying in its ineffective containment of the anxieties and fears about abandonment and death which abjection signals as waiting for us all, the final unknown.

Turning now to taboo, ignorance is

> ... epistemological alterity, tabooed epistemology, subjugated knowledge, or counter knowledge—the null curriculum of all that gets ignored, unattended, unacknowledged and left out of dominant conceptions of knowledge... [it] privileges certain paradigms of knowing as others are relegated to the realm of ignorance... even dangerous or evil.
>
> (Quinn 2011: 36)

A taboo is a socially set value or set of practices where substances, social practices and other matters are considered to represent a danger to a person or their health; or a societally determined understanding about what is pure; or defined as matter out of place (Freud 1955/1985; Douglas 2002). Taboo combines knowledge of what is sacred to us, as well as what is profane, uncanny, dangerous and forbidden (Freud 1955/1985: 71). This interweaving of the sacred with the profane in this one social construct is often overlooked when dealing with the kind of knowledge entrained into social learning about taboos and the associated rules and practices that sustain taboos' power to order our lives. Regarding taboos and their restrictions and prohibitions, Freud argues that the knowledge buttressing the setting of many taboos is lost in the past, with the result that taboos and their associated prohibitions become unquestioned practices for the social group. Moreover, while taboos set prohibitions and exclusions, they are not necessarily religious constructs coupled to an associated morality—wherein transgressors of taboos were thought to jeopardise their future and were considered polluted through their association with taboo objects or categories of people (Freud 1955/1985). Such a formulation has much more in common with Goffman's (1968) contemporary ideas concerning stigma and spoiled identity.

What is interesting about taboo and its role in managing potential dangers is how these categories, understood as taboo (objects, persons to be protected, polluting substances and so on), are attributed with uncanniness (unknown unknowns, weirdness) or destabilisation, even when much about the taboo object's dangerous status is unchallenged. Freud's concern with the role of taboo was linked more to the anxieties he had found expressed in illogical fears and neuroses or phobias that seemed to have similar mechanisms based in symbolism rather than reality, where a taboo seemed to stand in for possible pollution, rather than be based in a religious belief or actual fear associated with forbidden objects. Taboos, the uncanny, fearfulness and anxiety appear closely linked. In nursing and healthcare practices, they may be at the heart of food prohibitions (Meyer-Rochow 2009); contact with entities categorised as polluting, dirt or matter out of place (Douglas 2002); matters outside the boundaries of social propriety (such as discussions about death and, as discussed briefly in Chapter 3, sexuality); deviant activities; bodily by-products or excreta; bodies more generally; and any deviance that endangers 'normal' social interaction (Lawler 1991; Holmes et al. 2006b). Beliefs about what is taboo contain within them rules for appropriate social behaviour that nurses transgress in the routine processes of care; transgressions are often contained by 'traditions' and etiquettes of care. Hence nurses are located in dangerous places because the care they provide entails their breaching civilising social controls.

To many, dangerous ideas are those that contain some threat to the social order—they flirt with the epistemically treacherous. Sandra Harding (2006) provides us with an example showing how avoidance of danger contributes to ignorance. For many years, formal analytical philosophy has sustained a position against, and therefore ignored, specific theories claimed to be against the tenets of objectivity and disinterest. This, she claims, has led to an implicit bias within analytical philosophers' position. Harding proffers that such 'dangerous' theoretical perspectives (Marxism and Freudian psychoanalysis, for example) have been discredited because of long-held suspicions about the 'interestedness' of the theories and the conflicts with the received wisdom of American analytical philosophy. However, as Harding asserts, the two theories of interested ignorance put forward by Freud and Marx are discredited not purely for their internal problems (which others highlight while finding many of their insights useful), but because of the sociopolitical constraints engendered in American society as a response to the Cold War and the McCarthy era (Harding 2006). Understandably, scientists and academics have considered that use of these theories would affect their obtaining funding, or publication of their work. Staying away from such theoretical approaches amounted to strategic ignorance (Bailey 2007; McGoey 2012a), though not always acknowledged consciously. It also speaks to the self-censorship that continues to this day. It is obvious, too, that allowing that not all workings of the mind are available to us (due to the unconscious of Freud, or the false consciousness of Marx) was tantamount to acknowledging that not all was rational in the world of the mind—a situation that continues to confront those who hold to the privileging of Enlightenment beliefs about rationality as the dominant mode of thought (Sedgwick 2008).

But what has this to do with nursing and ignorance? Nursing developments in the mid-twentieth century were strongly affected by the constraints of academe in US universities. Dangerous knowledge such as Freudian and Marxian thought was cast aside in favour of Parsonian systems theory and other structural functional approaches to analysis, with an associated push for scientific theories of nursing and building of nursing knowledge. Moreover, in setting up such biased approaches to nursing knowledge, what emerged were theoretical approaches to nursing stripped of the murky realities of its practice base acknowledged by a psychoanalytic framework; a decentring and mistrust of the body (except as a cluster of symptoms and problems) and its associated (worrisome) emotions; or indeed any concern for how such sociopolitically-induced ignorance may have led to nursing's failure to confront the whiteness and inequities of the healthcare system in the USA (Barbee 1993). Not until after the 1960s and its emancipatory drivers was it possible for such dangerous thinking to be included in nursing's approach to its knowledge production (Allen 1985; Street 1990). Moreover, the shadows of the effects of denial of any forms of more radical thinking even reduced how nurses took up and used feminist approaches to build their knowledge. Such was the impact on nursing of conservative ideologies in academe (Kagan et al. 2014).

Abjection in healthcare work

As outlined above, abjection as an emotion evoked by, and an emotional defence against, horror is set early in our collective development. It resides in our bodies, with a reaction to horror that is both visceral and inarticulate. It is a reaction to commonplace fears, to the horrors of our uncivilised bodies as well as to our deaths. As an emotion, it overwhelms us with incomprehension, refuses rationality and waits behind, indeed, it may well be the motivation behind all the beliefs we summon to avoid thinking about our human frailty and unavoidable death. Nursing and healthcare work is located where the horrors of living are a constant. As an emotional state, very little time in nursing is put aside for thinking about what disconcerts us about nursing practices, and what work would make it possible for us to take seriously what is happening to nurses and patients when horror takes away our ability for 'rational' response. Recognition of abjection, on the other hand, exposes how our relationships with bodies and the bodies of others are necessarily fraught with uncertainty. This doubt may be a way into the productive use of the uncanny for an ethics of care that partially resolves our relations with bodily products, boundaries and practices that may be outside of what society considers clean and proper—and so perturbs us (Evans 2010). As well, such an ethic makes sense of the difficulties we have in communicating 'nursing' to others—too abjectly incomprehensible.

Our normative relations with the horrific are set to keep its visions at bay, to disavow, to misrecognise where or how nurses are located emotionally, to deny how this emotion is governing what we do, hence leaving much of this disturbing work unspoken (Alavi 2005). Nonetheless, as Kristeva and scholars of horror in cultural studies highlight, while the horrific repels and draws us equally and simultaneously, it remains unspoken. In so doing, nurses promulgate ignorance not only of their relations with their work, but also for and with patients as to what is happening when these emotions about our frail bodies threaten to overwhelm (Holmes et al. 2006b; Rudge 2009). A recent book deals explicitly with the abject and its play across the boundaries of the body, showing how abjection is about not illness, but states of disorder and chaos (Rudge and Holmes 2010). Schmied and Lupton (2010) assert that the chaos of a leaking body interferes with how a mother responds to breastfeeding, leading some to reject the experience in favour of the containment, 'cleanliness' and control of bottle-feeding their infant. Unless this is understood as a normal reaction to the lack of control in early feeding, many women cannot be supported. Nurses are required not to react to aspects of care that pass the containment of the civilised body, instead using sublimation as a containing explanation to the merely scientific—although, as we know from this book, such beliefs about the facticity of knowledge can only be transient: ignorance always lurks (Quested 2010; Roderick 2010). Moreover, bodily boundaries such as skin are overloaded with emotional import that is denied in science's approach to skin as mere covering (Gagnon 2010; Rudge 2015) or when body boundedness is transgressed (Holmes and Federman 2010). Nurses have to take account of behaviours that invoke anxieties about what is 'normal'. Here nurses are left dealing with deviant, illegal or betrayals of social norms such as familial or intimate partner violence (Bradbury-Jones and Taylor 2014). As McCabe (2010) highlights, nurses are rendered abject when they use nursing theories that fail to recognise how such knowledge is always incomplete—how it can exclude from 'normal' relationships and sexual activity those who are physically and intellectually different, rendering them abject.

The structures of the psyche frame how we deal with and deface (Latimer 2010) these early-learnt responses to the abject, and how this plays out when we are thrown into situations that horrify yet also fascinate. Kristeva (1982) identifies that science or religious beliefs are brought to bear on these dangerous knowledge(s) through their suppression of the possibilities of such dangers encroaching on nursing and healthcare activities. Aspects of abjection deal with matter out of place, just as taboos govern what is appropriate for discussion. Abjection lies unrecognised at the base of what we cannot, or will not, completely know, and what is characterised as horrific: betrayals or abandonments that destabilise our sense of normality.

Nursing taboos: openly secretive

While the actual mechanism underpinning taboos may be covered, (re)actions towards taboo stem from social norms; as Sedgwick (2008) terms it, they are open secrets. Discussion of taboos is necessary when we analyse accounts of ignorance in nursing and healthcare because of links to nurses' refusal to approach or care for 'taboo' groups (Beardwood and Kainer 2013) with certain stigmatised conditions, with spoiled identities, or who experience social discrimination based on moral concerns about their condition. Commonly in the literature, certain aspects such as particular conditions have been called nursing's 'last taboo' (Anon 1996; Burnard 1998; Freeman and Jaoudé 2007; McMillan 2008; Pearce 2012). These calls to address 'final' taboos are usually discussed in terms of effectiveness of treatment, nurses' anxieties about association with the condition, or how the condition is surrounded by social limitations, belief systems or rules that present nurses with difficulties in having open and frank discussions themselves or with their patients.

More centrally for this chapter, we ask: how does the social situation of taboo intersect with how knowledge and ignorance articulate in nursing?

Much of this discussion has to be extricated from papers where the notion of taboo is itself dealt with unproblematically—that is, merely opening up the taboo will lead to overcoming its troubling presence in nursing practice (Boyer 2011). As well, because these calls to address 'final' taboos speak to eradication of the suspect, erroneous thinking behind their continuation into nursing practice, the need to explore the relations between ignorance and anxieties about approaching changes is central. Moreover, nurses, positioned as they are as healthcare workers, are supposed to alleviate ignorance about taboo subjects for the layperson. Pinney (1979) suggests that changes in nursing or social care workers' attitudes to taboo cannot be successful without constant reinforcement of the necessary behavioural changes. Moreover, assumptions about how such change requires a single dose of an educational package underestimates how much work is needed to overcome beliefs held in common with the wider society. Our argument in this chapter suggests change also requires examination of the self, one's feelings, and nurses acknowledging how the abject figures in their responses to taboos.

Moreover, not only does the subject of taboo arise in situations that are set externally to nursing; there exist taboos set by nurses or by the organisation where they work (Roberts 2012) that, for example, suppress open discussion of the conditions of work through organisational pressures to not disclose certain situations. Many nurses must feel the pressure to not talk about service delivery matters, such as poor levels of quality in care, as systems promote silence and cover-ups. It is not a stretch to see that, given the pressures felt to be silent, there are taboos about what can be shared over and above the rules for confidentiality.

Many taboo subjects in nursing and healthcare focus on aspects such as psychosexual health and particular forms of sexual activities (for example, anal intercourse; disabled or child sexuality; or 'alternative' sexualities such as sadomasochism and transvestism); or on forms of violence such as intimate partner violence and sexual violence such as rape and child sexual abuse, all of which are bound by beliefs about relations between men and women, or the sanctity of the family. In some cultures, death and dying remain taboo topics. Notably, what counts as taboo has altered over time, and varies by settings as to what can be discussed properly (Walter 1991). Matters that were once considered taboo, such as homosexuality, are less likely now to be considered this way by all nurses, although not all cultural locations would allow nurses to have open conversations with their patients about all matters homosexual, bisexual or queer.

As many nursing authors have noted, such discussions remain silenced. Keighley (2012) points out, rightly, that subtle cultural understandings play into what should or should not be taboo, with westernised nursing often misapprehending how taboos affect nursing in other cultures. He highlights how in Japanese or Italian cultures, who knows and who can talk about an immanent death is very different from the purportedly open process in westernised countries. Moreover, what gets researched or seen as a social problem may overturn how we talk about social taboos in nursing and healthcare. What was formerly taboo may re-emerge as a topic of high social interest and importance when there is acknowledgment of the detrimental effects brought on by ignorance through historical stigmatisation and disparagement—something of the positive effects McGoey (2012b) reports as produced by ignorance. For example, research priorities for HIV/AIDS and breast cancer registered outstanding turnarounds in attention by governments after activist interventions by consumer rights groups in alliance with healthcare workers.

Open discussions about sexuality, bodily processes such as incontinence, stigmatised conditions such as treatment for HIV/AIDS (Gagnon 2010), or cancers such as bowel and lung cancer (Brown and Cataldo 2013), remain difficult. Many bodily processes remain taboo to speak about openly, just as the disgust engendered results in public controversy about the appropriateness of discussion. This may lead to the production of what Kempner and colleagues (2011) term 'non-knowledge'. Many taboo issues around body care emerge from the hidden work of nurses taking place 'behind the screens' (Lawler 1991; Gordon 2002). The operations of taboos and disgust lead to social ignorance about nurses' bodily care, which Lawler (1991) asserted led to devaluing of nursing care by both nurses and society. Indeed, body care and taboos surrounding bodily processes as matter out of place result in prohibitions about how to research bodies, thereby producing 'undone science' (Frickel et al. 2010) about body care and nursing practice (Ritchie 2013). Taboos resulting from abjection as matter out of place mean that nursing knowledge is sublimated into less controversial concepts associated with medical diseases, such as symptomology, intervention techniques, and scientific approaches to understanding experiences of illness through various tools and measurements (Rudge 1999). Interestingly, this has also led to a lack of work on embodiment in health and illness by nurses, as it is rare to explore such experiences through body work or body research (Lawler 2002; Picco et al. 2010; Schick Makaroff et al. 2013). This lack of contribution by nurses to research and literature on body work has meant a focus on this work as 'dirty', hence failing to challenge how this work is represented from a nursing perspective, and leaving body work in abject, taboo location—leaving it with the horrific, and not also as *jouissance*. Moreover, such failures can include studies of such body work where what nurses do to obtain the proper body of civilised society is not recorded in the paper (see Lawton 1998), making invisible not only nurses' organising work (Allen 2015), but the work most valued by people who need nursing care. This is not to discredit knowledge acquired through the lens of disease and measurement tools, which brought recognition of nursing research and care, but it becomes problematic when such research defaces patients' experience and nurses' work with bodies (Latimer 2010). We would argue that disavowal and sublimation of the entire experience of patients has an unknown impact on humanistic care.

Similarly, for many years, recognition of how emotions intersect in nursing as a result of the work was a taboo conversation, and certainly not something wherein the horrors of nursing work could be approached directly, as nurses were supposed to maintain distance and objectivity in their care (Alavi 2005; Evans 2010). In writing this book about ignorance, we are uncertain of its reception given the privileging of knowledge and the dominant conceptualisation of ignorance. We acknowledge that representing nurses as knowledge workers is a hard-fought position for the professional status of nurses in the healthcare hierarchy. As we work through the power of ignorance in nursing in this book, we hope to destabilise this taboo.

Other taboos in nursing are akin to the organisational taboos suggested by Roberts (2012). Organisations have practices that suppress knowledge, hide activities, record 'cherry-picked' matters, use statistical reports that fail to capture the extent of nursing's contribution. They do not keep all matters in the historical record, which contributes to organisational forgetting (Rudge 2003). All of this promotes ignorance of what accounts for nursing practice or other healthcare work (Latimer 2014; Allen 2015). It becomes a very partial record of what is valued at a specific time, but does not disclose all that occurs regardless of value. We will return to the effects of this form of silencing when we discuss how ignorance can be used or abused in the valuing of nurses' work by healthcare agencies, in Chapter 6. Where knowledge pertaining to the organisation of nurses and nursing is concerned, taboos and matter out of place play into what is suppressed, or indeed what is viewed as dangerous to know.

Dangerous knowledge as non-knowledge

As noted earlier in this chapter, the frameworks for thinking about ignorance (Barbee 1993; Harding 2006) emerge from theories of suspicion and negativity which continue to obtain purchase for the insights they can bring to professional education for healthcare workers, and to research on populations of interest by uncovering what remains unspoken, invisible and unremarked in mainstream accounts. What is ignored in such effacement of some theoretical approaches is that nurses encounter forms of knowledge and ignorance outside of what would be considered the norms for appropriate social or professional behaviour (Roberts 2012). Such actions mean that nurses negotiate the boundaries of ignorance in ways that result in disengagement from many challenging situations, as outlined above. Other forms of dangerous knowledge are also filtered out to maintain ignorance of particular patient situations (for instance, genetic findings from research; Lehtinen 2005). For example, information may be withheld from people on the grounds that such knowledge could lead to discrimination.

However, the idea of dangerous knowledge deals not only with forms of interested or strategic ignorance that deny or discredit local or specific knowledge. Dilemmas arise that are tied to disclosure of various knowledges: genetic inheritance (Takala 1999; Attard 2009), pre-implantation genetic testing (Rose 2005), the identity of organ recipients (Robertson-Malt 1998) and so on. What counts as dangerous is constructed according to 'unknowing', failing to recognise knowledge, or an 'ethics of best interest', all set by unquestioned social mores about gifts, who should know, and the social utility of the knowledge, against what will happen should such knowledge lead to exclusion from healthcare (Michael 1991). As mentioned in Chapters 2 and 3, abortifacients from colonising of the non-European world also constituted knowledge about women's control over reproduction, and such knowledge was discredited or censored in Europe, pushing the recorded properties of these plants, well known to socially disqualified 'healers' and 'witches', into oblivion (Douglas 2002; Schiebinger 2008). There are also censorship practices around disclosure of some behaviours such as suicide, where societal beliefs about taking life mediate the treatment of parasuicides (Morse 2001), the management/elucidation of unknown/misapprehended clues after the event (Bjerg 1967; Garfinkel 1967), and fears of copycat suicides (Rishel 2011). In participating in who is to know what and when, nurses actively and simultaneously produce, shape or shift zones of knowing and unknowing, strategically managing their patients, their care and themselves. This speaks to a particular ethics of the self around what is considered dangerous knowledge during the management of socially fraught questions such as: who should live, how people will die, who will have access to care, resulting in what Bourdieu (1977) terms complicitous silence. Dangerous discussion also revolve around controversies about nurses' involvement in situations such as the euthanasia programmes of the Nazi totalitarian government in Germany (Foth 2009; Benedict and Shields 2014); and the death penalty through lethal injections (Holmes and Federman 2003). Less controversially, and equally importantly to nursing, as Nelson (2009) highlights, there is the need to build histories that attest to nursing practices so as to overcome the historical amnesia resulting from the poor recording of what nurses do on a daily basis (D'Antonio 2006).

However, other forms of ignorance emerge in nursing due to how, at times, forms of knowledge are considered too dangerous, and the use of such knowledge is limited by traditional frameworks for nurses to think about their situation, their practice and their relations at/to work (Allen 1985; Harding 2006). Dangerous ideas are framed as such because they critique how we are to think about nursing, and they provide alternative perspectives considered to radicalise nurses' approach to their work (see Quinn 2011). Ideas and approaches such as feminism(s), critical analyses of many kinds, psychoanalytical theories, and postcolonial critiques of white domination in the global world of healthcare (Kagan et al. 2014) have all been marginalised from mainstream nursing research and knowledge production as a result of their discrediting.

With the introduction of neo-Marxist theorists such as Jurgen Habermas to the theorising of nursing research, practice-based approaches to knowledge production emerged that aimed to emancipate and empower nurses and their clientele (Street 1990). This in turn allowed dangerous critiques from women of colour to filter into nurses' approaches to research about its problem populations or vulnerable groups (Racine 2003). Dangerous knowledges that afforded critique found their ways into such nurses' publications as *Advances in Nursing Science* and *Nursing Inquiry*, and conference groups such as Perspectives on Feminist and Critical Theories in Nursing, as well as nursing philosophy and history conferences. The forms of interested ignorance are linked to subjugated and alternative forms of knowledge/non-knowledge based in epistemologies external to nursing. What these various fora allow is critical/ political discussions about feminism, psychoanalytic thought, bodies, Marxism, postcolonial resistance, class conflicts and discriminations and their power to maintain ignorance about the structural effects of class, gender, race and sexuality on nursing and its client groups (Barbee 1993; Van Herk et al. 2011; McKillop et al. 2013; see also Ahmed 2008; Malewski and Jaramillo 2011). Such thinking uncovers what is discredited or misapprehended to sustain nurses' ignorance of whiteness, gender blindness or the operation of discriminations in healthcare systems (Swendson and Windsor 1996; Latimer 1999; Puzan 2003). Moreover, what has assisted with this transition is the inclusion of many local knowledges, indigenous knowledges and acknowledgements of cultural specifics for nursing, as well as a gendered reception of knowns/unknowns that go against dominant or privileged accounts. Tied up with this form of unco- vering of ignorance is the concept of 'voice'. It recognises how multi-vocality avoids representing nursing with a singular, colonising voice that validates and legitimises many forms of ignorance, and that reproduces the *status quo* of nursing's relations with its clients and minimises heterogeneity within the nursing profession (Code 2008b; Quinn 2011).

Knowledge about what constitutes the social continues to be viewed as suspect knowledge because it presents pictures of society that might trouble healthcare professionals' privately held views, whereas blocking such knowledge limits how nurses can work politically for patients or other nurses. This lack of understanding of structures has led to ignorance based on nursing funda- mentalism (Rafferty 1995) and racialised features of healthcare and nurses' knowledge (Puzan 2003). Such ignorance has had a long-term effect on determining what knowledge is required for a practice profession. Without the critical discussions noted above, nurses risk remaining ignorant in *cul de sacs* or, worse, complacent in ghettos that do not make contact with knowledge/ignorance produced across disciplinary boundaries. As Tina Chanter describes it,

> thinking through locations where boundaries are less clear, where the mutual implication of structural issues such as class, race, gender or sexuality is more evident and none is given pre-eminence such as class or gender; where a body is predicated in parts, fragmented, its mean- ingfulness contingent; where we are in-between, unknown in terms of certain identities.
>
> (Chanter 2006: 92–93)

Conclusion

This chapter deals with ignorance in nursing where it intersects with social mores, emotions of disgust and horror, and dangerous knowledge. In each case, the situation presents nurses and other healthcare workers with the requirement to negotiate boundaries between what can be known and what comes to be suppressed or disavowed. In the case of abjection and taboos, we find that certain clinical conditions are girded by constraints, rules and understandings that get in the way of how nurses and other healthcare workers operate when dealing with taboo aspects of bodily contents or potentially polluted bodies, or when nurses have to talk about matters outside of normal propriety. Such situations are strongly affected by nurses' sociocultural setting. Moreover, what is viewed as taboo in one culture does not necessarily carry across to all nurses in all situations. Some situations, such as death and its rituals, vary according to religion and culture, yet nurses must have open communications about such matters. Nursing authors believe that overcoming societal barriers and having open discussions can lead to practices that circumvent socially set stigma, exclusions and marginalisations. Such breaking of silences caused by social taboos—such as confronting death, various sexual health conditions, or failures of bodily containments such as incontinence— also normalise nurses' work with bodies, thereby opening up their work for discussion, as well as challenging refusals to change that cause barriers to quality care for heavily marginalised client groups.

Ignorance and disavowal of knowledge are different for both abjection and dangerous knowledges where the problems rest with nurses' work and with society more widely. As Malewski and Jaramillo suggest in their conversation about ignorance, 'epistemologies of ignorance demand [we] attend to the production of unknowing and foreground exclusionary practices in understanding how dominant discourses are shaped' (2011: 4). In the case of taboos, uncanniness, and lack of acknowledgement of the effects of defences such as abjection around their work, nurses are required to do more than merely confront the situations; they must also act to show how such interests lead to maintenance and reproduction of what can be known in nursing and healthcare. Confronting what comes to be defined as dangerous knowledge requires nursing to challenge some closely held ignorances that have constrained and led to avoidant or poorly founded healthcare practices by nurses. Such exclusions of knowledge use require that nurses question what is dangerous, for whom, and in whose interests. How this form of ignorance relates to the politics of ignorance is explored in the next chapter. These understandings will then be used to explore how the uses or abuses of ignorance figure in, and are constitutive of, nursing and healthcare work.

5　The (bio)politics of ignorance

In making the case for the politics of ignorance, we must first recall that knowledge and ignorance, as epistemic transactions, are unequivocally matters of relationships (Townley 2011). In managing knowledge, one necessarily manages others. The same applies to ignorance: when dealing with ignorance, one necessarily transacts with individuals who ought to know, or who must not know. Nurses' and other healthcare providers' practice is precisely built around the strategic management of knowledge and ignorance in order to achieve health outcomes that are consistent with governmental objectives and priorities. In fact, at the core of 'health work' is the complex articulation of political rationalities and technologies pertaining to the government of subjects. By government, we mean the various modes of governance, including health governance, that encompass all aspects of human life; the political rationalities that provide such governance with substance and render it intelligible; the techniques of subjectivation involved, including by way of internalisation and self-government; and the modes of thinking and knowing upon which such governance rests. This approach is consistent with Michel Foucault's (1991) conceptualisation of governmentality and one of its core aspects, biopolitics (discussed below). However, it is worth noting that Foucault did not consider the importance of ignorance in these processes, as we intend to do.

Foucault heavily emphasised the way scientific knowledge (*savoir*) is at the core of government of individuals and populations. Such government is deployed at a distance, partly through the involvement of designated agents such as nurses, who mediate between state objectives and citizen subjects. It has been argued that nurses' proficiency in this regard rests on their power to engage in surveillance activities and to summon and activate various bodies of knowledge towards the betterment of individuals' and communities' health (Holmes and Gastaldo 2002; Perron et al. 2005). In this chapter, we wish to explore how nurses' management of ignorance, as well as the management of nurses' ignorance, plays an equally important role in that respect. Nursing practice can thus be understood as being grounded in social relationships resting on continuous epistemic transactions that hinge in large part on ignorance, uncertainty, incomplete information and provisional data. In exploring this idea, we examine the kinds of knowledge that are marshalled, or excluded, in order to formulate particular health discourses and therefore shape practices.

Immunisation programmes constitute useful examples for this discussion because their success depends on the circulation and uptake of specific knowledge, especially as it relates to infectious diseases and their management. Influenza immunisation campaigns provide particularly fertile ground for an exploration of the politics of ignorance, given the coordination of efforts deployed locally, regionally, nationally and internationally over the past decade to monitor and manage influenza prevalence and transmission. Immunisation programmes are also useful because they constitute a technology through which individuals can be governed in order to fulfil a state-defined health goal; nurses play a crucial role in ensuring the success of immunisation campaigns; and immunisation involves self-regulation to the extent that there is a strong normative expectation for citizens to endorse public health discourses regarding the risks posed by infectious diseases and to voluntarily submit themselves, or their children, to immunisation. Those who refuse are routinely castigated for failing to protect the health and safety of others; that is, as falling outside the (moral) norm.

Recognising self-regulation, for example in the form of acceptance and vaccination, as a core dimension of population health and management is consistent with a biopolitical perspective. Foucault (1978) described biopolitics as a core strategy of what he termed *biopower*, a rational mode of government committed to the protection, promotion and management of life. According to Foucault, biopower appeared throughout the eighteenth century in the Western world, as a modern response to a population surge which required new ways of preserving social order. As a form of power over life, biopower is concerned with all those elements that define, structure, strengthen, configure and enhance life. Foucault took care to specify that 'life', here, includes all aspects that make up the social, such as activities, discourses and practices that enable one's participation in the public realm and one's connection to fellow citizens and the state; but he also emphasised biological life as a pivotal area of concern. In his view, biopower involves 'the set of mechanisms through which the basic biological features of the human species became the object of a political strategy, of a general strategy of power' (Foucault 2007: 1). Through biopower, biology as it underlies the minute processes of life thus falls within the realm of politics. Health and illness are therefore key features of how one is to characterise one's life, but also of the way one is to be governed in society.

Biopower involves a range of strategies, techniques and agents aimed at organising, monitoring, governing and optimising life. Anatomo-politics is concerned with managing the individual, while biopolitics focuses on the regulation of the collective body (Foucault 2007).

> The objects of biopolitics are not singular human beings but their biological features measured and aggregated on the level of populations. (…) [It] refers to the emergence of a specific political knowledge and new disciplines such as statistics, demography, epidemiology, and biology. These

> disciplines make it possible to analyse processes of life on the level of popu-
> lations and to govern individuals and collectives by practices of correction,
> exclusion, normalization, disciplining, therapeutics, and optimization.
>
> (Lemke 2011: 5)

Following Foucault's analysis, we can posit that the management of health risks such as contagious illnesses falls within the realm of biopolitics: first, because it is concerned directly with a biological condition that determines where one fits along a health–illness (or life–death) continuum; second, because it connects with a range of interrelated disciplines (microbiology, physiology, virology, epidemiology) that systematise and supply the expertise necessary to comprehend the phenomenon at hand; and third, because it sets in motion a range of discourses, technologies and bodies of knowledge aimed at categorising the condition (and, in this case, the pathogen responsible for it), and managing it. For example, patients who present at hospitals for influenza-related symptoms and complications may have samples collected that will undergo laboratory testing to confirm the source of infection. These samples may then be sent to a designated influenza sentinel centre that collects such samples and other data about infected patients (prior vaccination, complications, etc.), maintains a pathogen database and a 'flu activity' map, and collaborates with other authorities (regional, international e.g. WHO) in the coordinated efforts to monitor, respond to, prevent and contain flu outbreaks. Statistics, projections, recommendations and policies then flow back to health agencies worldwide to provide representations that are as accurate as possible of the prevalence of influenza, patterns of contagion, morbidity and mortality rates, which strains predominate, their antigenic properties, and so on. What is of particular interest for our discussion is the calculated and synchronised deployment of con-siderable efforts to manage problematic realms of knowledge and ignorance inherent in biopolitical operations such as the identification, containment and management of infectious diseases such as influenza. As mentioned earlier, we also have a particular interest in the way nurses are deployed in order to ensure the success of these operations.

Regulating biologies: from viruses to citizens

Because of their close work with individuals and communities, nurses are ideally positioned in such endeavours—and to perpetuate certain types of ignorance and knowledge that may otherwise be contested in scientific and clinical circles. Nurses' epistemic labour is grounded in biopolitical rationalities to the extent that, in order to carry out effective health interventions, they must collect knowledge about the individuals and communities they care for, for example in the form of assessment interviews and risk appraisals, collecting information such as a person's weight, immunisation records, family history of heart or liver disease, breastfeeding practices, smoking habits, and so on. They must also examine patients' knowledge levels to determine whether an educational intervention is warranted (e.g. teaching about immunisation or healthy eating). Nurses working in this way probe the scope of patients' knowledge and ignorance as these play out *vis-à-vis* their bodies and their biologies. Part of nurses' role is to teach patients about (and dispel their ignorance of) how to care for themselves, by imparting knowledge on various conditions and prevention methods or treatments. Patients become self-aware as they learn to recognise lacunae in their own knowledge, identify a pattern of problems in their health practices, and align these with nurses' instructions. Coercion is unnecessary: compliance is secured because patients voluntarily partake in the improvement of their health outcomes by disclosing much information about themselves and then by espousing nurses' teachings. Partnerships such as these between healthcare providers and patients are effective because they uphold the subject as a rational, autonomous, sovereign agent. Nurses can thus normalise individuals' understandings according to current health policies as well as promote desirable lifestyle and treatment choices (Perron et al. 2005). Through such normalisation, nurses actively construct patient subjectivities (Holmes and Gastaldo 2002). This, however, begins with the proper flow of knowledge: patients become effective self-regulating subjects first and foremost because they become both *knowable* subjects and *knowing* subjects.

In the management of pathogenic transmission, and by generating significant bodies of knowledge on health issues, state and public health officials engage in biopolitical strategies aimed at harnessing collective energies and wills toward the safeguarding of an identified health concern that affects a significant proportion of individuals—an outbreak, one of the figures of catastrophe. Nurses play a pivotal role in this regard. For example, they are thought to be well positioned to improve vaccination rates (Lau et al. 2012). The expectation is that nurses can address patients' concerns and convey information that is favourable to behaviour modification (e.g. immunisation) in order to comply with public health recommendations. As seen earlier, nurses' expertise and their ability to obtain information about their patients are key in achieving this goal:

> Nurses need to use their knowledge and consultation skills to understand relevant aspects of health psychology and to apply them in a therapeutic manner. Health professionals must elicit their patients' ideas, concerns and expectations about this immunisation, and be prepared to mount a respectful challenge, not only for at-risk patients but also with our colleagues if they decline vaccination.
>
> (Warner 2012: 27).

The epistemic labour involved in biopolitical goals is therefore quite clear. And though Warner makes no mention of ignorance *per se*, it is clear that ignorance is at play in the interactions she describes. Those whose thinking and actions do not align with normative claims and standards therefore embody paradoxical subjectivities that govern how credibility judgements about them are made.

First, they are varyingly valued as *informants* (credible testifiers) or as *sources of information* (passive suppliers) (Fricker 2007, in Code 2008a). Second, they oscillate between *autonomous experts* of their own body, experiences and needs, and as *ignorant subjects* in the face of science and technology innovation, healthcare administration, vaccination technique and public policy. Objective or subjective knowledge collected from patients is thus integrated within the discourses of nursing, medicine, public health and epidemiology.

In our view, health agents' epistemic labour in the context of biopolitics, however, takes on another form: the management of ignorance through a problematic knowledge base. As Foucault argued, biopolitics rests in large part on the organisation of knowledge, for example as described earlier regarding patient knowledge. However, this can also be understood as the formal organisation of a corpus of knowledge that unifies, centralises and governs particular epistemic discourses and practices in recognised disciplines such as virology, immunology and epidemiology. Nurses enjoy considerable authority with patients, in part because their practice rests on credible sources of knowledge, particularly what has come to be known as 'scientific knowledge'. In the context of influenza immunisation, however, it is worthwhile to explore the making of this formal knowledge further.

The problem of the virus

Influenza is described as a highly infectious, acute respiratory illness. Once known simply as 'the flu', something prompting ample rest and fluids during cold winter days, it has become established over the past decades as a life-threatening disease carrying a high rate of hospitalisation, complication and mortality, and requiring careful monitoring and management in order to contain its spread amongst a population. According to WHO (2014), annual epidemics of seasonal influenza alone may amount to 3 to 5 million cases and about 250 000 to 500 000 deaths. Whether in its seasonal or pandemic form, influenza is no longer confined to the bedroom of the coughing and aching individual. It is a matter of public risk, biosecurity and economic burden, and as such it spurs a wide and synchronised range of activities in order to contain its spread and effects. Such efforts are visible, for example, through the extensive and ramified activities of the WHO Global Influenza Surveillance and Response System (GISRS), which is responsible for monitoring the evolution of influenza viruses and potential mutations, assessing risks, and making recommendations about vaccine composition, based on samples received from designated National Influenza Centres across the world. This work is assisted by research laboratories and institutes worldwide dedicated to the understanding of the complex behaviour of influenza viruses, and peer-reviewed journals are replete with articles presenting the latest findings. Influenza research and management rests on the deployment of an extensive collaboration and communication network—that is, it gives rise to a distinct epistemic community (Townley 2011) in which knowledge (and lack thereof) is generated, transmitted and administered in a systematic manner. It is a true exercise geared toward the management of ignorance in the form of uncertainties, as these networks attempt to forecast the behaviour of viruses that mutate from season to season (a moving target), and whose genetic and clinical features cannot be fully known until an outbreak.

National influenza campaigns worldwide rely on information provided by the GISRS and medical scientists regarding influenza epidemiology, risk groups, and trends in transmission. Health policies around influenza management generally aim at intervening at the individual and population levels in an organised and systematic, though voluntary, manner. Influenza immunisation campaigns, deployed in many parts of the world, have worked to organise citizens in a non-coercive fashion, with varying levels of success. Various associations and coalitions have developed to support these campaigns, such as the Canadian Coalition for Immunization Awareness and Promotion, Influenza Foundations in Thailand, India and Indonesia, and Influenza Specialist Groups in Australia and New Zealand. These entities are often a mix of professional, government and private sector representatives. Their goal is to envision and realise creative campaign strategies aimed at furthering the goals and effectiveness of national and regional vaccination programmes. This is achieved through the publication of brochures, promotional videos, pamphlets and posters, as well as the organisation of educational sessions, all of which disseminate the key messages of immunisation programmes: mainly that influenza can have deadly consequences, and that protecting oneself helps protect others. Such messages entail a logical course of action in the form of getting vaccinated.

Such undertakings effectively mobilise the interests and capacities of multiple stakeholders with key messages about the need for, and benefits of, risk-based health initiatives, and the responsibilisation of all of those involved, not just lay individuals, but health practitioners as well. For example, Canada's National Advisory Committee on Immunization (NACI 2012: 36) makes the moral duty of health professionals very clear in this regard: 'In the absence of con-traindications, refusal of HCWs [healthcare workers] who have direct patient contact to be immunized against influenza implies failure in their duty of care to patients.' Such statements typically rely on various health studies, clinical/experimental research findings, consumer surveys, economic impact studies and cost–benefit analyses that are presented as converging toward similar conclusions about the overall benefits of mass influenza immunisation. These assessments, in their own way, help to render a complex issue—viral pathogenicity in humans—intelligible or, in Miller and Rose's (2008: 62) term, 'thinkable'. They constitute the knowledge base necessary to make immunisation, and the solicitation of citizens, a worthy, reasonable and accepted state objective.

Miller and Rose point out, however, that health programmes such as immunisation campaigns are not 'simply formulations of wishes and inten-tions' (2008: 62). In order to be coherent and accepted, they must mobilise particular bodies of knowledge about the issue at hand, such as the health of populations and, more specifically, the elderly, pregnant women and children, those whose health is deemed to be compromised because of pathological processes (e.g. immunocompromised patients), or those who experience chronic states of vulnerability (e.g. individuals of lower socioeconomic status). They call out to the population (and, in the case of influenza immunisation, those who care for them) by conjuring up medicalised understandings of common ailments, moral responsibility and self-efficacy. Economic arguments constitute an important aspect of these campaigns; however, they are brought into the equation chiefly to explain the economic burden of disease, in the form of loss of productivity and work absenteeism. On the other hand, other economic considerations, such as market imperatives as a catalyst for such campaigns, are often absent. Central to the activation of immunisation campaigns are the relationships effectively tying the individual and the collective, the abstract and the concrete, the present (e.g. current knowledge and understandings) and the future (e.g. interpretations of potential risks). Influenza is no mere disease. It carries its own organising capacity of time, space and subjectivities well outside the realms of the clinic and its associated disciplines (e.g. virology). It also powerfully ties citizen bodies to the collective and its political, institutional, disciplinary and economic contingencies.

Viruses interact closely with the social; so too does science (Latour 2004). Scientific information stemming from clinical trial data helps to establish a normative position regarding the way we manage viruses and vaccines. And there is no doubt as to how sceptics should be treated. For example, commenting on the measles vaccine, Armstrong (2015), editor of the *Medical Journal of Australia*, notes that '[t]hese latest battles in the "vaccine wars" are in some ways encouraging: the voice of scientific reason has received widespread coverage and community backing, while the anti-vaccinationists have been shamed'. Armstrong's view is rather common and contributes to widespread censorship and ostracising in the name of science. However—while one may find comfort in the optimistic view lauding science's capacity to support social phenomena and progress through the generation of sound, objective knowledge— in the context of influenza immunisation and treatment, scientific foundations are less sturdy and clear-cut than originally thought. For example, several researchers from the authoritative Cochrane Collaboration have called into question the effectiveness of influenza vaccines, identifying it as 'modest' at best (especially in populations aged 65 and higher), and as rapidly decreasing as time passes. They also challenge the view that the vaccine is effective in preventing influenza, transmitting influenza, and preventing complications (Jefferson et al. 2010a, b; Osterholm et al. 2012; Jiménez-Jorge et al. 2013; Thomas et al. 2013; Demicheli et al. 2014). As a result, the benefits of mass influenza immunisation are put in doubt because of the costs involved in relation to their effectiveness (see e.g. Simonsen et al. 2005; Jefferson et al. 2008, 2010a, b; Schabas and Rau 2015; Skowronski et al. 2015). Other studies have reached similar conclusions in relation to neuroaminidase inhibitors, antivirals that are used to treat influenza (Cochrane Collaboration and BMJ 2014; Jefferson et al. 2014a). And others have highlighted the selective reporting of findings or the conflicts of interest that appear to influence accurate portrayal of the benefits and risks of the compounds used to manage both seasonal and pandemic influenza (Cohen and Carter 2010; Dunn et al. 2014; Jefferson et al. 2014b; McCarthy 2014; Lenzer 2015), leaving important effectiveness and safety information in the dark and thereby maintaining uncertainty and ignorance in that aspect.

Surprisingly, in this era of evidence-based medicine, there has been very limited, if any, uptake of these analyses in contemporary public health discourses, despite the fact that they have been conducted using what are deemed to be the most rigorous research methods: systematic reviews, meta-analyses and randomised controlled trials, as opposed to, say, observational studies. Perhaps such results can be likened to a form of dangerous knowledge in the tightly regulated space of influenza discourse, because of their potential to challenge the status quo and because they provide arguments to 'vaccine resisters'. Following these various publications, policies in the USA or the UK, for example, remained unchanged (CDC 2012; Torjesen 2014). Nursing organisations do not relay these publications to their members. And it appears as though binary 'pro' and 'con' positions have hardened. Science, as the foundation for evidence-based practice, is serving all sides of the discussion: rigorous studies are proposed to establish definitive narratives about influenza, immunisation and other modes of infection transmission containment (such as wearing a surgical mask); the overall conclusions of these studies have been challenged, as seen above, notably by the Cochrane group; and so too its own analyses have been problematized (e.g. BCCDC 2013). Influenza is both an overdetermined and an underdetermined object. Overdetermined because, as an object of ongoing concern and inquiry, it is defined equally through epidemiological, organisational, bureaucratic, economic and ethical terms, thereby saturating everyday discourses about health, safety, risk, responsibility and accountability. Yet at the same time it remains underdetermined because of the range of contestations it breeds, whether at a scientific, social or ethical level. It does not matter whether such contestations are considered to be absurd, valid or, perhaps, conceivable. What matters is that they also suffuse a number of discussions in lay and specialised circles. Regardless, what remains clear is that public health campaigns, and the support (or contestation) they generate constitute powerful organisers of citizens' collective consciousness by aligning interests and energies. Converging and diverging views regarding influenza immunisation are expressed by health officials, patient advocacy groups, lay individuals, media reporters and scientists. Multiple subjects therefore partake in a sustained (and often fierce) debate to establish what is 'true' and 'accurate' about influenza and influenza immunisation—in other words, a struggle for epistemic legitimacy.

On nurses', and others', knowledge and ignorance in the context of influenza

More and more organisations require their health workforce to be vaccinated and, because healthcare workers' vaccination rates remain modest, many advocates push for mandatory immunisation (Poland and Tucker 2012). In some cases, this has led to loss of employment by personnel refusing immunisation, despite philosophical or religious objections. In nursing, discussions about these issues centre mostly on the ethics of immunisation: regularities in discourses characterise nursing organisations' pronouncements regarding the need for healthcare workers to be vaccinated in order to protect patients (e.g. ANA 2010; CNA 2012; ICN 2013). This lends an interesting dimension to the notion of nurses using their self and their body as a 'therapeutic tool' in order to care for their patients. In this case, a vaccinated body is thought of as providing safety and reassurance, as serving as an example for hesitant patients, and as safeguarding the flow of care against a burdensome illness (ICN 2013).

It has been suggested that if healthcare workers do not endorse influenza immunisation, their ability to educate or influence patients is likely to be reduced. Indeed, whether working in schools, hospital settings, long-term care facilities or community clinics, nurses can play an important role in relaying to patients the latest information released by public health agencies, in educating patients about the benefits and risks of influenza and its vaccine, and therefore in improving patient vaccination rates. They can do so first by generating an interest, a desire that becomes subjects' own. Subjects can then 'rationally calculate their own life risks' (Lemke 2011: 49). That is, nurses are in a good position to supplement or correct (normalise) patient knowledge and bring about a modification in behaviour towards the optimisation of their health and their life. As seen earlier, this is a central aspect of the biopolitics of healthcare work.

While patient knowledge is clearly identified as a site of intervention, so too are nurses' knowledge, attitudes and disposition to accept prevailing discourses regarding influenza immunisation. However, these discourses make no mention of differing views among scientists regarding its rationality and cost-effectiveness. And while nursing unions and organisations have generally taken a stance against the compulsory immunisation of healthcare workers (with some exceptions, e.g. College and Association of Registered Nurses of Alberta 2014), such positions commonly rest on the detrimental effects of coercion on a workforce, and nurses' right to autonomy and bodily integrity (Sullivan 2009; CFNU 2012), rather than nurses' understanding of the conflicting evidence regarding influenza immunisation effectiveness.

Because of their knowledge of infectious processes and concern with patient wellbeing, nurses should 'naturally' be favourable to immunisation, including their own. A lack of endorsement constitutes an anomaly in the expected configuration of attitudes towards this public health intervention, and, as seen in the quotation above (NACI 2012: 36), it elicits questions about these nurses' moral agency. Unsurprisingly, critics of nursing organisations who do not support mandatory healthcare worker immunisation conjure up longstanding values of duty and selflessness to challenge such positions:

> one would have hoped that the data would trump anecdote and reason trump misperceptions (...) upholding nursing's historical and important

role as advocates for patient safety, fulfilling the ethical tenets of the healing professions where self-effacement and service in the interests and well being of the patients they are privileged to care for dictates behavior and policy.

(Poland and Tucker 2012, 1754)

Nurses' refusal to vaccinate has also prompted hostile reactions from members of the public denouncing nurses' selfishness and unprofessionalism, and it has been suggested that such a stance is detrimental to the credibility of nursing as a profession (Poland and Tucker 2012).

Knowledge and reason remain at the heart of the matter—or so it seems. In exploring the reasons why many nurses decline influenza vaccination, various researchers cite nurses' erroneous knowledge or beliefs about the vaccine, for example regarding its effectiveness (Toronto and Mullaney 2010). Others, however, simply frame nurses' ability to use reason and logic as faulty. For example, McGeer (2013) makes the following unencumbered statement about unvaccinated care providers, including nurses:

> these providers feel that the risk of influenza vaccine is greater than the risk of not being protected against influenza. It is that 'feeling' that may be at the root of the problem. Neuroscience now tells us that strong feelings of fearfulness are the natural human response to risk... our brains are hard-wired to pay much more attention to immediate feelings of fear and much less attention to the evidence about the actual levels of risk... There is good evidence that the human emotional response to risk sometimes results in poor decisions. We need to recognize the risks associated with these emotional responses as they apply to vaccines... It is thus particularly important that we don't allow emotional responses to override the evidence when making decisions about influenza vaccination.

This statement was published in *Canadian Nurse*, a journal published by the Canadian Nurses Association (CNA), and it generated strong critique—not from a nursing organisation, but from nurses themselves. These nurses responded to McGeer's contention by underscoring nurses' use of scientific evidence (such as a Cochrane review published by Thomas et al. 2013), by calling out McGeer's own objectivity in light of her undisclosed ties with the pharmaceutical industry, and by calling for scientific studies that are free from pharmaceutical influence[1] (Ballard et al. 2013). The view of nurses as 'feeling' rather than 'reasoning' is particularly pervasive in professional and public circles (see Ceci 2004 for a compelling example). This perpetuates ignorance about the kind(s) of knowledge used by nurses, all the while portraying them as ignorant of current scientific advances. Those who fail to accept the 'right information' cannot, therefore, be recognised as credible knowers, even when their reasoning is based on what would normally count as rigorous scientific evidence—that is, when they adhere to the rules of epistemic and scientific legitimacy.

Those who work in the field of influenza research, policy and prevention face a difficult task, one that, ultimately, is one of government: government of knowledge, attitudes and practices (including 'bodily practices' such as vaccination and other protective techniques e.g. hand washing, coughing in one's sleeve) against the behaviour of an uncertainty-laden pathogen. This governance also serves to manage gaps in research and policy, and secure the necessary monopoly over circulating influenza discourses. Such concerns are all the more amplified in the case of a pandemic (Davis et al. 2013). Epistemic communities such as those discussed earlier produce guidance, based on past and current information, toward the management of indeterminate futures. Regulating individual and collective biologies is a key aspect of this endeavour. Ignorance in the form of uncertainty; unknowns (what Mansnerus 2014: 80 refers to as the 'silence of evidence'); omission (through selective publication of trial data, e.g. Every-Palmer and Howick 2014); and dismissal (the overlooking or rejection of conflicting scientific information) help define the biopolitical objectives of public health's efforts in regulating minds and bodies. Sick and healthy bodies alike are the discursive objects in this case. In fact, healthy bodies are equally problematic from a public health point of view because they may propagate infection unbeknownst to the unsuspecting carriers. Healthy bodies, or what are thought to be healthy bodies, are therefore equally risky, unruly, and in need of prophylactic 'discipline', toward the productive goal of maintaining the health of populations. This government occurs through specific epistemic lines where those not formally recognised as 'knowers' are required to trust and endorse expert discourses (Perron et al. 2005).

As such, while we deeply value Foucault's (1978; 1991) argument regarding the central role of knowledge in governmentality, we suggest that the anxious desire to govern individuals and aggregates subjected to everyday life processes stems in larger part from the unknowns attached to these processes and to the limits of scientific inquiry. Citizen bodies, with their complex and often unpredictable biologies, are an object of study, categorisation, discourse and intervention. Their unknowns, much like their (possibly provisional) knowns, constitute an object of government. Bodies make possible the mobilisation, transaction and enactment of various discourses and practices. Self-government, for example through the uptake of vaccination, is enacted because of its hoped-for protective features in the face of ever-changing and unpredictable viral mutations and transmission patterns. The self-governing subject can thus be depicted as a sovereign, rational and responsible agent, but we argue that s/he is first and foremost an anxious agent who must exercise caution and demonstrate foresight in the face of insecure futures. Self-governance, put simply, rests on ignorance, an ignorance that lends the required authority to harness resources, mobilise energies, and act in particular sanctioned ways. Bodies-at-risk therefore provide opportunities to enact agency. This, however, does not boil down to a simple matter of cognition. As seen earlier, affective elements (e.g. feelings of vulnerability, sense of responsibility) are mobilised towards the effective implementation of technologies of government, including self-regulation;

they are also helpful in the assignment of blame in case of failed self-responsibility and accountability, regardless of motivation. In other words, ignorance has the power to organise, and it shapes discourses and subjectivities accordingly. As seen earlier, patients and healthcare providers alike are simultaneously subjects and objects in these knowledge and ignorance transactions, and both are subjected to categorisation as reasonable or unreasonable knowers, depending in large part on their acquiescence with dominant discourses. In the pursuit toward 'ideal' knowledge, knowledge can become an instrument of ideology and thereby generate a range of practices that can produce various forms of ignorance.

Conclusion

Influenza research and management in the face of uncertainty is a useful example to begin exploring the multiple and conflicting ways in which presumptions of knowledge and ignorance shape public policy as well as citizen behaviours. In the ongoing debates about public health interventions, such as immunisation and post-exposure prophylaxis, social, political and epistemic negotiations take place that have particular individualising and collectivising implications. Of course, the case of influenza is just one, very current example among many suitable for this discussion, where we can productively link ignorance to the management of everyday life. Ignorance adds a revitalising angle to an analysis of the biopolitical administration of risks, as a necessary precondition to, and feature of, particular modes of (health) governance and subjectification: first because it works to identify areas of health 'non-knowledge' that need correcting; and second because it perpetuates further ignorance if the inconsistencies in the body of science used for health education remain concealed.

Risk and uncertainty are conflated, and 'science' is their most potent answer. Yet, as Haraway (1989: 3) argues, '"Science says" is represented as a univocal language.' It is often portrayed as

> indisputable speech, a previously invisible form of political and scientific life that made it possible sometimes to transform mute things into 'speaking facts,' and sometimes to make speaking subjects mute by requiring them to bow down before nondiscussable matters of fact.
>
> (Latour 2004: 63)

We will return to this issue of science and research practices in Chapter 6. In the meantime, however, it is important to note that refusal to engage with the continuous interactions between science and the social blunts the possibility of exploring the productive effects of ignorance beyond understandings of ignorance as a mere catalyst for scientific discoveries. It therefore maintains more ignorance about the crucial role that ignorance, in its multiple manifestations, plays in shaping human experiences, or about the ways it configures liabilities of thinking, knowing and acting in relation to identified collective concerns. As Proctor contends (2008: 26), '[d]ecisions of what kind of knowledge "we" want to support are also decisions about what kinds of ignorance should remain in place'. And these decisions are not a matter of intractable laws of nature, but of the weaving of complex epistemic agencies and power relations that configure how 'we' are to think and act in the face of unknown futures. The scientific, the clinical, the epistemic and the political are therefore tightly bound, and, as seen in the renewed debates about influenza, attempting to isolate these realms from one another constitutes a rather futile endeavour. Importantly, it may also constitute an attempt to sidestep the (bio)politics of ignorance and its role in everyday biological and social life.

Note

1 Aside from the reality that much of contemporary influenza research is funded by industry, or is conducted by scientists and physicians who have ties to industry, it is worth noting also that many of the influenza coalitions mentioned above also receive funding from the manufacturers of the vaccines and antivirals they promote.

6 Ignorance in nursing

Its uses and abuses

In this chapter, our argument is based on the twinning of the two concepts of knowledge and ignorance. As states of knowing, or even 'being', as we have traced in previous chapters, knowledge and ignorance exist together, in relation. As McGoey (2012a) asserts, ignorance is knowledge, and we have argued throughout this book that what builds knowledge requires attention to ignorance. We began this book detailing how errors, neglectful care and scapegoating operate to reduce ignorance or error to discussions about ethics, the legal/regulatory and/or ethical issues of whistleblowing, and explorations of systemic conditions that deny culpabilities. We showed how using 'ignorance' and its workings to explore what are indeed systemic issues helps interrogate how culpabilities are assigned and how power works throughout to displace blame and challenge the maintenance of the status quo; as well as to indicate how, if ignorance is not brought to the equation, the situation continues without benefit in the future.

Nursing has been reliant traditionally on medical knowledge to build its own knowledge base, that is, knowledge necessary to support nursing practice and education. Interestingly, in medicine and healthcare in general, ignorance is discussed very narrowly using a pragmatic view of what we do not know and what we should know, building programmes of research to cast ignorance aside. In medicine, Duncan and Weston-Smith (1984) provide an excellent example of this matter-of-fact approach. Tremendous efforts have gone into delineating the boundaries of nursing knowledge, extricating what is unique about it and how it differs from more established disciplines such as medicine and psychology. There is, however, no consensus over what this knowledge is, or whether it even exists. There seems to be a general opinion that nurses have a unique way to generate and handle knowledge, putting what is known to work to provide tailored care to individuals in times of need.

Classic texts, such as Carper (1978) (with subsequent revisions by White (1995) and Munhall (1993) about sociopolitical knowledge and 'unknowing', respectively), have outlined how nurses know, and what shapes that knowing (Berragan 1998). Since the 1950s, nursing scholars have deliberated on what nursing knowledge is, how nurses practise using that knowledge, and how it underpins nursing's position in the healthcare system (see Donaldson and

Crowley 1978; Robinson and Vaughan 1992; Barnum 1998; Rafferty 1996; Meleis 2012; Reed and Shearer 2012, and numerous others each addressing matters of nursing ontology and epistemology in their own way).

The focus is on expanding knowledge, building 'nursing's knowledge base'—clearly there are theoretical, philosophical, professional and, as has been argued elsewhere, political implications as well. Among calls to build, construct or affirm nursing's knowledge base, there were nurses who contributed to what we would term exploring the realms of ignorance in nursing (see previous chapters for much of this work). We also explored how ignorance is used as a form of deception, denial or containment of dangerous ideas so as to not have open discussions about disconcerting issues, such as nurses' role in the holocaust in Nazi Germany (Foth 2009); roles in racist and colonialist practices (Ramsden 1990; McKillop et al. 2013) and how they may take part in regimes of punishment and state killing through death penalties (Holmes and Federman 2003). All of these controversies are examples of the interplay between knowledge and ignorance cloaked by secrecy, shame and moralities of ignorance that position nurses working in these situations on the right and wrong sides of societal debates about human rights, racial discrimination, capital punishment and other dangerous/controversial ideas.

In this final chapter exploring the politics of ignorance in nursing, our attention rests on an exploration of how the politics of ignorance plays out in the arena of building knowledge—and simultaneously how ignorance can be used and abused in the process. As we have shown throughout this book, the picture is complex because what could be thought of as an abuse of ignorance in nursing from one perspective, could be explained as useful for nursing in its desire for control over its future developments and thinking. We have chosen to undertake this through an exploration of a specific set of operations that play into knowledge development in nursing. These epistemic and practice activities are concentrated in research to obtain evidence for practice; concerns about ensuring that nurses in all clinical settings know how to access and use such research; and ways to evaluate how changes to practice are implemented and bring improvements in quality and safety, as well as feeding into nurse education.

This complex set of activities is interwoven into what we see as an apparatus of knowledge and/or ignorance in nursing. Each aspect involves a conceptual understanding about nursing, in the process surfacing how and what nursing knows. Rather than focusing merely on knowledge, we are going to explore how the various actions contribute to, promote and maintain ignorance in terms of how nurses (and probably many other healthcare workers) understand or misunderstand their position in contemporary healthcare systems. In each area (research practices, knowledge use, auditing) we explore how certain epistemic positions use or abuse ignorance in their processes. Finally, we explore a subjectivity available for nurses that offers a way to use what they do not or perhaps cannot ever know as a way to centre nursing and its practices. We explore epistemic agency, and how the politics of ignorance results in a multiplicity of positions within the epistemic community of nursing where collaborative models of care and 'response-ability' (Latimer and Munro, 2015) result without depoliticising the insights derived from ignorance. Being response-able requires nurses to question, rather than rush to solutions that deprive themselves or their patients of epistemic agency in healthcare systems.

The politics of ignorance and research practices in nursing and healthcare

> Science is always wrong (…) It never solves a problem without creating ten more.
> George Bernard Shaw (October 28 1930)

Science has long been, and continues to be, thought to provide valuable and reliable answers to the subjects of scientific research. Yet, as George Bernard Shaw noticed, answers routinely open up further questions unanswered or problems unsolved. As Stuart Firestein (2012) notes in his beguilingly small book entitled *Ignorance: How it Drives Science*, we all want to be seen as knowledgeable and not ignorant. In exploring the research practices of nursing, we believe many directions towards which nursing knowledge development is going are fuelled by Firestein's insights about the place of ignorance in science. In his exploration of ignorance and the practices of science and knowledge production, he makes a strong argument for the view that science starts where facts run out (Firestein 2012: 12). He further asserts that what is truly mysterious, ignorance, is growing rather than diminishing in the face of our race to know and use all we know—in defiance of what we do not know about what we know. Firestein locates our limitless ignorance in how much we know now and how little we know of the available knowledge in our information-rich societies (though this can be debated since few have access to information). In his view, the interface between 'facts [that] serve mainly to access ignorance' [are the fuel for science that] 'traffics in ignorance, cultivates it, is driven by it (2012: 15). Nonetheless, what he regrets is that we still have too many answers, or at least we put too much stock in answers. This emphasis has 'produced a warped view of science' (16). Instead, he argues for a science that views its central activity being about 'ignorance generation' (18). More centrally to a book about ignorance, as the aphorism goes, data is not information, information is not knowledge, knowledge is not wisdom.

Firestein's view strongly supports the idea that research, and practices that support it, are based at the edge of what is known and what we do not know—the unknown (see also Smithson 2008). However, we have practices based on understandings about evidence which may not be in the zone between ignorance and what we know. Instead, they may lie in the zone that Kleinman and Suryanarayanan (2102: 509) term 'normatively induced ignorance', wherein normatively set ways of undertaking research lead to knowledge from one point of view, or decontextualised questions and results without strong relevance to clinical contexts. The focus on evidence-based practice has led to the use of randomised controlled trials (RCTs) or other methods that suffer from reductive questions, paradigmatic purity, and failure to provide research that informs nursing interventions and speaks to conditions and complexities found in clinical settings. Such situations mean that research risks being irrelevant to patients' situations (Cartwright 2007).

The division of epistemic labour is also apparent in the way proponents of evidence-based medicine (EBM) and developers of best practice guidelines (BPGs) assume a powerful knowing role over those who do not know, or are assumed not to know because they do not appear to know the 'right' thing, that is, the received evidence on which to base their clinical practice. As is widely known, the hierarchy of evidence originally put forth by the Canadian Task Force on the Periodic Health Examination (1979), and updated a decade later by Sackett (1989), the Evidence-Based Medicine Working Group (EBMWG) and the Cochrane Collaboration, purports to eliminate unreliable expert opinion, promoting instead the uptake of evidence derived from meta-analyses, systematic reviews and RCTs. It is interesting, however, that eminent proponents of EBM, such as the EBMWG, the Cochrane Collaboration and the Joanna Briggs Institute[1] (JBI) (Pearson *et al.* 2005), do support the training of 'EBM experts' or 'champions' so as to facilitate the integration of high-ranking evidentiary sources into clinical practice. This implies that there are different categories of experts where EBP is concerned, and that authoritative groups such as those mentioned here stipulate the terms under which proper expertise can be recognised as such.

As a consequence, epistemic agency is redefined through EBM, with its focus on the generation, appraisal, acquisition and utilisation of appropriate, relevant knowledge. This has implications for the division of epistemic labour, to the extent that new, restructured roles are put forth for the researcher, the clinician, the patient and the policy-maker, yet the subjectivity of such agency for nurses is rendered irrelevant. In the first fifteen years of the movement, the development of scientific knowledge appeared as a neutral, pure and value-free endeavour, devoid of subjective content (Goldenberg 2009). However, traditional scientific approaches conceal the fact that knowledge, skills and technology are borrowed from multiple cultures and are multi-authored. This obscuring and forgetting of patterns of origins promotes systematic ignorance (Conner 2005). Relying on relevance guidance, which is enshrined in normatively set ways of evaluating knowledge (through knowledge utilisation or knowledge users), leads to suppression of knowledge about either the context or local knowledges, or about the way the research does not, in fact, have relevance in the local setting (Kleinman and Suryanarayanan 2012).

Moreover, in selecting or framing knowledge in strictly utilitarian ways, what we have is many areas of 'undone science' where research that might have had broader application or utility is unfunded, and so not done because it will not lead to a successful research/academic career or promotion (Frickel et al. 2010). So, in thinking about knowledge and ignorance and the use of knowledge (and perhaps more importantly the use of ignorance), what becomes apparent when one interrogates the situation of ignorance is that questions require to be privileged above answers; that spaces between the facts might be more central to our understanding than the facts themselves (Firestein 2012: 20).

In the next section we outline the kinds of legitimacy gained, and what is at stake when we consider the consequences of the power of ignorance (Kleinman and Suryanarayanan 2012), where epistemic privileging 'institutionalize[s] particular kinds of ignorance' (494)—say, about effectiveness of nursing interventions or implementation of BPGs—and values some evidence over others 'in different professional and intellectual fields of practice' (495). As highlighted above, social and epistemic production of ignorance follows particular routes. In healthcare, the problem of ignorance in relation to research practices highlights how, due to the confluences of legitimacy, timing, problem definition and weight of opinion, the result is dominance of some forms of research, and the sidelining and marginalisation of specific forms of research, the knowledge obtained from them and the dismissal of alternative knowledge—'the upshot is ignorance' (497).

As Cartwright (2007) suggests, the RCT process is closed to the many forms of the unknown in how both treatment and outcome are operationalised. The ignorance produced in this political economy of research knowledge production consists of non-knowledge—producing false knowledge (Smithson 1985); it leads to a situation of undoable research, or research that is undone because the case for alternative views is rejected. For instance, Kleinman and Suryanarayanan (2012) assert that 'by not considering inconclusive results worthy of legitimate consideration, researchers prefer a variety of ignorance to a variety of knowledge' (508), that is, '*normatively induced ignorance*' (509, emphasis in original). In their exploration of bee-keeping science, they show how the field of bee science favoured hard data 'over bee-keeper "anecdotes"' (509). They assert that the result was undone science, compounded by research that did not actually reflect the dynamic settings of bees and colony collapse disorder, which in turn 'distort[ed] subsequent knowledge *and* non-knowledge production' (510, emphasis in original). As regards bee toxicology research, the effects of epistemic privilege turned the research gaze away from the contextually sound knowledge of bee-keepers. For example, it privileged the claims of agrochemical companies which asserted that their newer, low-toxicity products were safe for use by farmers, based on research using deliberately shortened cycles. This disallowed research into the possible long-term use of low-toxicity products, thus obscuring the concerns of bee-keepers. Such politics of ignorance is not unknown in bioscientific research: use of pharmaceutical products in healthcare, and finance sector economics, are two forms of research where similar strategies play out (see McGoey 2012b; Davies and McGoey 2014). In nursing, the use of RCTs in complex clinical and social situations runs up against similar issues (Lindsay 2004). We suggest that nurses attempting to apply such research to practice are not unlike the bee-keepers trying to maintain bee health in the face of research that is not 'open to unanticipated events and to uncontrollable and context-sensitive settings' (Kleinman and Suryanarayanan 2012: 501).

Knowledge utilisation and the eradication of ignorance?

Since ancient times, when Socrates thought about what it was 'to know', we have questioned how much more there is to know, how little we know, and how much we live in ignorance. Indeed, Socratic questioning and other pedagogical approaches rely on the privileging of questions and the maintenance of ignorance to create an active learning subject who finds their own answers rather than those provided by a 'teacher' (Keller and Keller 2011). From one perspective, then, the promotion of knowledge as 'useable' is useful to nursing in light of calls to use select research evidence—as exemplified by EBN and the promotion of evidence on which to base nursing practice, rather than tradition, rituals or routine. We will explore how the industry of knowledge utilisation (KU), promulgated to prevent ignorance, uses ignorance as an argument for its promotion in healthcare settings. We outline what the approach has achieved, and we explore KU's abuse of ignorance. We argue that a closer inspection of KU reveals a politics of ignorance that results in less productive forms of ignorance that are embedded within its practices. Though KU focuses on gaps and tardiness in new knowledge uptake, it fails to evaluate the social dimensions of the context, and the limits or incompleteness of the knowledge produced.

First, we explore how epistemologies of ignorance play a part in critical analyses of what counts as knowledge. We want to move away from the rather naïve assumptions about ignorance that underpin the KU industry in healthcare. We ponder how to develop an ignorance utilisation perspective that goes beyond ignorance as mere absence or void or, worse, unused knowledge due to non-compliant or actively resistant end-users. Healthcare research is dominated by similar forms of normatively set procedures, with large profitable companies undertaking health research, profit-driven pharmaceutical companies, and academic practices all instituting a set of assumptions about what counts as legitimate knowledge, that works to produce ignorance as much as to provide knowledge. Therefore how ignorance is promulgated by an industry developed to promote knowledge use is germane. Our intention is not to diminish the work many nurses have undertaken to research nursing situations and care clienteles, but to highlight the epistemic contingencies of such endeavours. We do not wish to review the entire KU movement. Rather, we will explore how this new 'science' may be about 'the dying bee' as much as it is about ensuring health practitioners' research uptake towards improvement of standards of care.

Nurses are often blamed for being resistant to change, for hindering the implementation of new practices (Jutel 2008; Bail et al. 2009; Beardwood and Kainer 2013). Such nurses are perceived as 'old school', ignorant, unscientific, unprofessional and unethical. Nurses do resist some forms of change, perhaps because, despite reassuring and enthusiastic championing, their experience tells them that the new practices seldom yield better patient outcomes but often corrupt care environments. Through experience, nurses develop strong skills that support their practice with individual patients, but that have none-theless been negatively portrayed as mere 'habits' or 'traditions'. Nursing struggles still with accusations of using pseudo-science as a strong driver of the profession, or of its research activities (e.g. Johnson 1999). Those who embrace non-positivist approaches, in the form of postmodern analyses or qualitative research, for example, are a prime target for criticism and ridicule, typically by positivist purists grounded in disciplines such as epidemiology and the so-called hard sciences (see e.g. Sokal and Bricmont 1998; Goldacre 2006; Sokal 2006).

As stated in our discussion of taboo, the influence of traditions in nursing is disparaged extensively by researchers and leaders in nursing and other dis-ciplines, in colourfully worded articles such as Gibbs and Gambrill (2002), Rauen et al. (2008), AACN (2014) and Makic et al. (2014). These authors specifically refer to ignorance and tradition as barriers to the 'conscientious, explicit, and judicious' use of best evidence as promoted by Sackett and colleagues (1996). Such approaches leave no room for discussion or counter-arguments challenging the highly deterministic, eurocentrist and overly optimistic discourses surrounding evidence-based practice (Charlton and Miles 1998; Miles et al. 2008; Miller and Miller 2011; Every-Palmer and Howick 2014). It is worth noting, however, that the original intent of EBP has been profoundly distorted: in about two decades, the call to assess and use evidence *in conjunction with clinical judgment and expertise* has been reinter-preted as resting exclusively on the so-called gold standard of research, the RCT. Nurses do not have a tradition of RCTs in their practice, but they do have a tradition of trial-and-error and empirical observations to explore clinical and organisational issues (Rankin 2009; Urban 2014).

Ignorance in the framing of KU is viewed as having dire consequences for continuous improvements in care, better health outcomes and cost-effectiveness of care. It is the negative of positive knowledge, a vacant space requiring filling with available knowledge, through the application of knowledge about KU. Several issues drive this movement, located in the problem of 'solving social problems with knowledge' (Estabrooks et al. 2008: 50). This is not so different from Firestein's (2012) perspective on how ignorance drives scientific research to produce better health, patient outcomes and sound clinical care; or the finding of a solution to the theory–practice gap, or as Estabrooks et al. (2008: 53) put it, the 'know–do gap'. Sound KU evaluation requires interrogation of the characteristics of the knowledge user, survey of the stakeholders in the research, and estimations of the relevance of the research to their use (Graham et al. 2006). The field grew out of the need to ensure funded research was used to achieve increased productivity in agriculture, and its other influences are thought to be various races to knowledge such as arms, space and the need to manage economic competition (Estabrooks et al. 2008: 51). The movement is also inextricably linked with safety and cost-effectiveness in healthcare. Hence research utilisation and the broader concept of KU are strongly situated in a utilitarian framework without much consideration for what knowledge is, what counts as use, and the strongly normative agenda of the ethics of knowledge use.

If we explore how knowledge is conceptualised in KU, or the assumptions underpinning its activities, we have to acknowledge that KU is consumed with the facts to erase ignorance. However, if we view KU through the lens of ignorance, we see how it is peddling ignorance where knowledge is over-valued in relation to ignorance or its utilisation as 'facts'. As Firestein (2012: 21–22) suggests, facts are never trustworthy; claims to facticity and knowledge are valid for only a limited time before such facts are untrue, or less likely to be true.

Looking at KU and its presumptions, the qualities of ignorance are ignored in favour of a naïve belief in the completeness and certainty of the science that underpins treatments, guidelines, protocols and the like. Yet KU under-estimates how scientific work 'proceeds in fits and starts of ignorance' (Fire-stein 2012: 22). It cannot account for the continual shortcomings emphasised in the many reports investigating failings of the healthcare system, as outlined in our introduction; or for the provisional or experimental nature of medical treatments, set by guidelines and protocols that are insufficient, based on incomplete knowledge—a form of ignorance production that remains neglected in safety and quality discourses.

Knowledge utilisation aims to ensure that nurses apply knowledge to clinical practice through the application of implementation science about KU. However, it is possible that the knowledge about the causes of ill health may be producing more ignorance (and, indeed, more illness). Unreliable data are presented as uncontestable facts through statistical relationships. Limits to knowledge and limits to ignorance rely not on what could be known, but rather on what is currently appraised in terms of utility. As with the bees, the scientific practices that have set up knowledge production in medicine were instituted by research processes that are biased towards *normatively induced ignorance* at best, and false knowledge at worst. Blinding is therefore not only blinding for control, but also to the ignorance produced by and through scientific methods used to prove clinical outcomes (Cartwright 2007). Nurses' resistance to research use may be because the practice setting destabilises the certainties promised by KU discourses (Rayner 2012).

Audit culture as a centre of ignorance in nursing

This chapter now turns to an analysis of how audit culture (Strathern 2000) operates to use or abuse ignorance in nursing. Audits are performed to evaluate the implementation of guidelines, clinical pathways and other nursing inter-ventions. Audits are part of the apparatus of calculation to promote efficiencies and effective practices in healthcare organisations, and linked to research practices, KU programmes into the localised culture—audit culture. Moreover, calls for auditing of clinical nursing turn the lens away from what may be inducing a sense of uncertainty in nursing practices, focusing instead on accounting for what happens and making this visible.

The use of the audit and its associated culture is linked to other elements we have explored in this book. Nurses in many clinical settings use the framework of audit to prove the effectiveness of their nursing practice, to legitimise their effectiveness to the healthcare system—a remarkable yet persistent form of ignorance about a large part of the healthcare workforce. Audits are thought to ensure acknowledgement of the work nurses do within this framework, which is built from accountability structures that have been dislocated from audits' original focus (see Strathern 2000). This ignorance that fuels efforts by nurses to validate their role also relies on the perspective that 'healthcare' is hospital-centric and dominated by budgetary constraints and productivity issues (Blakemore 2009). Other matters include requirements by government to ensure clinical safety (Garling 2008), safe hospitals (Heartfield 2002), and risk management (Reith 2004). Nurses' consent to audit is manufactured through a focus on rendering nursing visible in the calculations of the audit (Burston et al. 2011; O'Neill et al. 2011; Allen 2015). What matters, rightly, in the development of in-depth nursing knowledge gets obscured in validation activities of the audit, leaving nurses in a state of ignorance as to what the audit actually accomplishes. When nurses' knowledgeable work is ignored by non-recognition in the audit, unfortunately work that is most valuable to the organisation is privileged, and its value is hidden to the worker (Thurlow and Jaworski 2012; Allen 2015).

In healthcare, much like the wider capitalist system, its economic system is governed by rules and strategies similar to those of production systems more legitimately aligned with capitalist rules for production. Moreover, as part of these challenges, clinical safety and high-quality practice are sentinels of the health of this system; they require forms of research that ensure accurate pathways to achieve accountability and processes for clinical governance that can be calculated 'objectively' (Miller 1991). As seen earlier with KU, knowledge development is linked to the role it plays in safety and security, having little to do with the health conditions of the population, or the state of the healthcare system in many countries in the world. In the audit cultures of hospitals, nurses' work is timed in information systems used to track patients through the system; in nurses' care planning, timings of protocols are set in the system and then used to predict staffing needs; and all this timing is used to calculate patients' time in the system from admission through to discharge and perhaps beyond. When times are set that re-design nurses' work, urgency, intensification of work practices and a focus on health service requirements mean that practitioners are not able to give time to those things that counted formerly (Rudge 2011).

The hope of the technology of the audit is precisely its ability to count activities and to reassure that everything has been done, and also can be *seen* to be done—as seen earlier in the introduction with regard to governmental inquiries. Underpinned by rationalities and calculations (more or less statistical), the audit is viewed as a way of obtaining information which can guide the standardisation of efforts, and obtain efficiencies and safety as well as quality improvements in clinical practices (Davies and McGoey 2014). With the rise of audit culture, Strathern (2000: 2) observes how the idea of 'audit' has been cut loose from 'its moorings in finance and accounting; its own expanded presence gives it the power of a descriptor seemingly applicable to all kinds of reckonings, evaluations and measurements'. She notes that the audit takes up time for development of processes and forms of assessment, taking resources (material and human) away from direct work—work that is forming what counts. It curtails nursing research as being about efficient and effective care above all else (Berragan 1998). Research in the clinic is considered of little relevance unless it has direct clinical import as defined by its use of a narrow range of activities, such as protocols, guidelines and clinical pathways (Barnes and Rudge 2005; Rankin 2009). Increasingly, nurses' clinical research is governed by medical and scientific paradigms, or domesticated through EBN (Holmes et al. 2006a) or practice development (Rudge et al. 2011), excluding the possibility of critique (Rankin 2009). As Kipnis (2008: 282) asserts, the new bureaucrats, central to the management of the contemporary bureaucracy, 'use [forms of audit] either because they see them as effective in local social contexts or because their superiors demand they do so'.

The application of audit technology to estimate nursing effectiveness, through the amplification of knowledge and visibility, requires to be understood, therefore the articulation of ignorance and invisibility in the process of audit must be unpacked. Recalling the scandals highlighted at the beginning of this book, we can see how audit techniques have reinforced the need to measure more, or better, or to regulate more firmly to avoid such situations. In audit culture, the impetus is to do better with the audit, leaving the examination of the processes of audit and its limitless production of ignorance outside of examination, and therefore 'unlimitedly productive' (see Davis and McGoey 2014: 79). In such a situation, audits and the culture surrounding them have deeply contradictory impulses embedded in their strategies—what we see as counter-strategies that reinforce audit's failure to predict the unknowns that develop in healthcare bureaucracies, where knowledge is always already incomplete.

> The codification of new rules following a corporate scandal is that knowledge generally becomes more expert and more inscrutable, and therefore less accessible or accountable. Yet, paradoxically, through the launch of yet another inquiry or through the introduction of new rules, *the illusion* of transparency is strengthened, and individuals sigh in relief over the observation that at least something is being done.
>
> (McGoey 2007: 219; emphasis added)

Despite the ongoing failure of the apparatus of audit, outlined above, the abuse of ignorance continues when management and executives of healthcare bureaucracies claim ignorance about certain situations. Alvesson and Spicer (2012) claim an analysis of stupidity is more useful than managerial theory, which focuses on learning organisations as the pinnacle of organisational strength. Rather, they assert that 'functional stupidity' (2012: 1196) is as important if not more so than smartness for the smooth running of systems, through standardisation, protocols and guidelines that allow for unthoughtful activities. However, ignorance does not necessarily imply stupidity—either of an organisation, or of the people who manage it. Sedgwick's (2008: 7) conceptualisation of the relations between power and ignorance suggests how not knowing resists knowledge, particularly when 'obtuseness itself arms the powerful against its enemies'. The difficulty arises when employees, customers, and those trying to work out who is accountable or responsible are figured as 'enemies' (Roberts 2012). Ignorance is produced to hide power, disguise power, blind us to who is accountable, while nurses are kept busy obtaining evidence of how well the system runs. How can ignorance work in their favour?

Agency developed in this way does not deprive the other of their epistemic agency. It speaks to the epistemic condition that we are all ignorant with incomplete knowledge, particularly when some of that knowledge is categorised as expertise. This stops nurses and other healthcare workers from falling into the trap of assumptions about what 'we think we know but do not' (Kerwin 1993: 180). Such an argument has implications for how we approach uncertainty in healthcare, where many practices put in place to 'manage' its presence result in the promotion and maintenance of many forms of blindness. As Croissant outlines,

> Someone somewhere knows something, someone elsewhere does not. Someone knows there is something to be known. That which is to be known may be based on probability or stochastic processes which have a residual uncertainty. These knowings and non-knowings are not patternless, but neither are they completely specified or structured.
>
> (Croissant 2014: 7)

Rather than unknowing what we know so that we can find out more by questioning patients or clients (Munhall 1993), a way is opened where questions rather than solutions are privileged. This reflects McLaren's (2011: xiii) call for us 'to be strategic outsiders, and tactical insiders' because, like education systems worldwide, we in healthcare face similar major changes which aim to privatise/re-industrialise health using utilitarian modalities such as neorationalism and neocolonialism. We are witness to the effects of reduced health budgets peddled as necessary solutions (Moody 2011). We are double-blinded in advanced capitalist economies to the strategic ignorance of governments as they deny real effects of 'reforms' while our gaze is taken from the disasters to count and count again in the failed systems of the audit culture.

Conclusion

The problem that comes with the rush to solutions we decide from mis-understanding that ignorance and knowledge are in a binary relation (Code 2004) is that such 'mishandled ignorance can be more costly, harder to perceive, and so harder to correct, ... hence limiting rather than liberating' (Firestein 2012: 39, 45) us with new knowledge. Structures that sustain ignorance (and knowledge) are understood too crudely through utilitarian and neorationalist schemas of research production and KU that do not engage with the complexities of ignorance and its strategic use in advanced neoliberalism. Clearly, scientific methods, social structures (race, gender, class etc.) and academic practices are reified by ignorance and continue to hide the work of all workers and organisers of healthcare (Thurlow and Jaworski 2012). If we interrogate knowledge through the workings of ignorance, we have 'ecological questions, and the responsibility imperatives, both epistemic and moral—invoked by ignorance' (Code 2014: 301).

If we can state 'I don't know' with a sense of its power, we question the utility of knowing everything, the privileging of solutions resting on false knowledge, and listen to what is said by those in between, subjects of both ignorance and knowledge, open to both use and abuse. The perception of use and abuse is often dependent on where you stand on knowledge development. It is our contention that health research and its knowledge use, Others' bodies, and the 'populations' they constitute are healthcare researchers' *terra nullius*. The unknown is set structurally through levels of strategic ignorance and epistemic privilege where ignorance is misrepresented yet embedded in what we know and the ways in which we choose to chase knowledge. As with the science of knowledge, where we seek control and predictability, even contextual research is accomplished through tools and measurement, reported as variability, yet objectified through use of psychometric tools that maintain ignorance. We remain ignorant of how privileged knowledges or positions sustain the very structuring of knowledge and ignorance as non-recognition, non-science, undone science, and discrediting of the right not to know. Epistemic agency and responsibility, trust and ignorance, are key to how we live and work with what we do not know and perhaps cannot ever know. Surfacing ignorance has implications for how we practise, educate or research within nursing settings as widely dispersed as academe and clinical or educational settings.

Note

1 From its inception, the JBI has attempted to have a broad definition of research to include in its reviews, and to this end, many reviews include meta-synthesis of qualitative research. Such syntheses are, the authors note, more than summaries, and so include interpretation of the collated papers and re-presentation of qualitative data (Pearson 2010).

7   Conclusion

It is not possible in a book of this size to cover everything about ignorance and its manifold articulations. One of the challenges lies in first developing a comprehensive and definitive portrait of the way ignorance has been handled so far as a specific focus of inquiry, or as only one part of broader social phenomena, and then drawing this literature into, and rendering it intelligible for, academic and professional disciplines in the health domain. Throughout this book, we have endeavoured to introduce the rich concept of ignorance into health and nursing scholarship. That is, we have tried to make ignorance 'thinkable' (Miller and Rose 2008) in nursing and healthcare, not only in negative terms, not only as a lack of knowledge, education, or science, but also in positive and productive ways, as something that makes the social 'work'.

And so it is clear from our analyses that we cannot limit our understanding of ignorance as something that can simply be resolved with more education. Education as an emancipatory and empowering strategy may be quite limited in contexts where ignorance is, or must be, strategically and productively deployed. Promoting education as a straightforward answer reiterates a view of ignorance as an individual trait, as always detrimental, and as a void requiring that we simply 'add knowledge and stir'. As seen in Chapter 5, implementing educational strategies may simply mean abating ignorance in some areas of cognition while maintaining ignorance in others, which can only enable the expression of a subject's agency in a particular predetermined direction that may, in fact, not be in the subject's best interest. Of course, we are not denying the value of education or emancipatory approaches but one should always ask: emancipation from what? Towards what? Involving, but also *excluding*, which kinds of knowledge? Asking such questions with ignorance as a starting point may lead to revitalised problematisations of prevailing discourses of power, autonomy, freedom and knowledge (whether developed through education or research).

In this book, we touch on how ignorance cannot always be replaced with certain knowledge—yet this does not stop busyness in nursing to attempt what is difficult and perhaps nigh impossible to do, that is, eradicate uncertainties. Some aspects of nurses' work, such as disgust and abjection, lie outside civilised social conversations: we have argued for the various ways nurses' means of controlling uncertainty and emotional anxieties, often unconsciously. How these uncertainties feed into nurses' responses to their lives remains outside current, mainstream 'thinking' about nursing. We show how many forms of knowledge are avoided in favour of those aspects believed to bring control over the uncontrollable. Dangerous ideas that destabilise certainties required by and cultivated through managerialist imperatives, including clinical guidelines, protocols for 'safe' practice and other measures for 'effective' nursing, are defaced and ignored. Nevertheless, such ideas and emotions escape the guards commonly put in place.

Constructing nursing as objectively known denies the rich veins of emotion guiding nurses' work, often outside of conscious thought, outside the 'body sciences' that fail to address the realities of body work. Social or psychoanalytical understandings of illness remain outside mainstream 'clinical' research, outside the reassuring construction of guidelines. Scientific management is privileged epistemically in most evaluations of nursing, for example under the aegis of audit culture. Audit's problematic knowledge-building deprives nursing of knowledge about its work, producing non-knowledge instead. As stated in Chapter 6, such misdirected research amplifies the urge to measure, rather than attempt different approaches outside the certainties of scientific management. Indeed, the certainties hoped for through scientific research and management accelerate rates of uncertainty about the meanings, significance and status that nurses ascribe to and derive from their work.

Knowledge development is, of course, a worthwhile endeavour. Though often comforting, knowledge is only ever provisional, as argued by Firestein (2012) and many others. Critique, as we see it, is a powerful part of this process of identifying the shortcomings, the limits, the shadows of knowledge. But any research endeavour beginning with a hypothesis, or setting out to prove or disprove a theory, is engaged in such a venture. Many authors agree that knowledge only breeds more ignorance. We agree with this stance to the extent that knowledge often leads to more questions and uncertainty. Yet we take this point further and suggest that more knowledge also breeds more ignorance through more *opportunities* for such knowledge to be resisted, doubted, countered, denied, censored, overtaken or forgotten (for example as was seen with tobacco research, see Proctor 2008, and again currently with climate science). This brings on more calls for more knowledge in a never-ending loop. In order to investigate such dynamics, analyses grounded in epistemology (and in particular feminist epistemology), sociology and philosophy are indispensable.

Diversifying analytical perspective makes it easier to problematise those uninterrupted discourses that promise to 'improve care'. For decades, nurses have been enrolled in various trends, including nursing theories, nursing diagnoses, clinical pathways, evidence-based practice, practice development, rounding and Lean Six Sigma—'simple' remedies for such complex issues as human experiences and behaviour. These have possibly brought some benefits to care, but have also created quagmires of contradictions, uncertainty and failed promises, particularly when these tools appear to care better for organisations than for patients or providers. As such, they can generate bias, ambiguity, indeterminacy and a sense of irresolvability.

Many nurses candidly endorse these tools, not realising perhaps that they rest on epistemic privilege and have built in them rhetorical devices that actually devalue nurses' experiential knowledge and exclude them as credible knowers. When these approaches fail to deliver on their promise of better care, the blame often shifts to nurses, while ignorance is maintained about the misguidedness of overmanagement through instruments that always remain grounded in bureaucracy and techno-rationality. Such maintenance of ignorance has violent effects. It maintains nurses as scapegoats in the system; it alienates nurses from their own empirical and intuitive knowledge; and it leaves nurses with the epistemic labour of reconciling discordant knowledges resting on differing paradigms, realities and agencies.

These approaches can also be violent for patients, to the extent that they situate them as precarious knowers in organisations. That is, they are said to promote patient experiences and expertise, all the while subjecting them to knowledge produced remotely from their daily realities as patients. Such approaches also promote changes that often overburden care (e.g. through added bureaucracy, staff cuts) thereby increasing burnout, accidents, morbidity and mortality. And while knowledge-building apparatuses such as research, inquests and public commissions may appear to be patient-centred and focused on transparent, unbiased and systematic fact-finding, they routinely help maintain strategic ignorance through selective questioning, investigation, reporting or follow-through, which protects those in managerialist positions who, through unconscious or wilful ignorance, refuse to engage with messy (Schön 1988) human and social realities, and thus perpetuates the status quo.

We contend that the bulk of issues encountered in healthcare settings are, in fact, not 'clinical' at all. They are first and foremost epistemological issues and, more specifically, issues related to the epistemic division of labour, the associated construction of particular subjectivities (that are valued or devalued), and the power relationships that govern these configurations. Dismissing the relationship between knowledge and power, and therefore ignorance and power, (re)produces a particular kind of ignorant discourse. We have already touched on issues of power as they relate to knowledge and ignorance. Along with Code (2008a,b, 2013, 2014), Townley (2011) and Vitebsky (1993), we agree that ignorance is not so much the absence of knowledge, but rather evidence of the confrontation between different forms of local knowledges culminating with the domination of some forms over others. The political implications of Vitebsky's observation are therefore clear when he states that 'knowledge and ignorance, then, are not so much cognitive as evaluative terms' (1993: 101).

And so, while it is tempting to think that relying on 'sound' and 'proper' scientific evidence is a foolproof strategy to sidestep these problems, such strategy is certainly naïve and possibly misguided. As Hulme (2007) argues, 'The danger of a "normal" reading of science is that it assumes science can first find truth, then speak truth to power, and that truth-based policy will then follow.' Given the multiple and opaque processes that govern the way only certain scientific facts are published, receive credence and ultimately shape policy, it is clear that ignorance is not just a fertile ground for scientific discovery, but a productive entity, socially constituted to facilitate health governance in specific, state-sanctioned directions, towards what are deemed to be productive outcomes (Kleinman and Suryanarayanan 2012; McGoey 2012b).

In the health domain, prying open spaces of ignorance and examining the involvement of particular professionals such as nurses in its operations is a complex undertaking. However, we believe it speaks to the level of maturity of a profession willing to self-analyse and to critique the way it is made an object or a subject (in a Foucauldian sense) in the politics of health. For instance, it is often thought that nurses can operate as ethical agents, or maintain a discourse as such, only if the power relationships pervading their practice remain overlooked or ignored, and if their practice continues to be discursively constructed as neutral, patient-centred and scientific. Nurses' close involvement with individuals and communities makes them strategic (biopolitical) agents in knowledge configurations in which knowledge about, say, patients' health and behaviours is carefully collected and categorised, while state-produced normative discourses (regarding who is healthy, ill or at risk, what parameters are used to produce these categories, and how to manage them) permeate nursing work and shape citizens' practices.

Nursing practice is a (bio)political practice because it governs the life (and death) experiences of social aggregates. Nurses tend to understand and interpret their practice as 'clinical work'—that is, work grounded in the clinical realm. Foucault (1978) shows how the modern understanding of the term 'clinical' is highly problematic; how it obscures processes grounded in the social, the political and the ethical; how it is saturated with power relationships that assign meaning, value and significance to certain things and certain subject categories, and not others; and how it obscures the processes by and through which these assignments are made. As seen throughout this book, nurses and other health professionals must strategically manage realms of knowledge as much as realms of ignorance. In conveying only specific information about specific issues, they maintain ignorance that has broad implications for the legitimacy and sustainability of state- and professionally sanctioned health education and policy formulation. Scientific inquiry, professional practice, and practices of the self (in the form of self-regulation) articulate with each other at the juncture where knowledge and ignorance meet.

Nurses constitute an epistemic community insofar as much, if not all, of their work revolves around the acquiring, handling and transmission of knowledge: for instance, learning new procedures or policies, participation in research rounds, documentation of patients' subjective accounts, completion of risk assessments (e.g. patient falls, violence or suicide), handover of patient assignments, and teaching of self-care techniques, to name just those few. These activities all require knowledge management, but also ignorance management—nurse ignorance, organisational ignorance, patient ignorance. Nurses are enrolled in epistemic communities interacting with other epistemic communities that inform their practice and whose discourses (e.g. evidence-based or vocational approaches to nursing), practices and knowledge they integrate and internalise, in large part by keeping uncertainty and the abject at bay. Enrolment in productivity programmes provides nurses with seemingly certain and supportive knowledge—only to have such certainties broached with the next patient, the next crisis, the next scandal, and avoidance of engaging with what nurses' work actually involves. Perspectives on the distribution of ignorance through any system offer the possibility to eschew culpability (Code 2014), yet also indicate how ignorance is limitless, productive and multiform.

Nursing scholarship discusses such issues to an extent, but this remains inconsistent, and analyses tend to be confined to specific constructs, such as professional competence and excellence, patient safety, decision-making, bioethics, or patient–nurse collaboration. As seen in Chapter 6, structures of nursing knowledge development encourage narrow areas that are researchable by nurses, and they restrict appreciation of what 'clinical' represents and of how barriers to 'knowing' are constituted in the research and managerial cultures promulgated in health and research bureaucracies (McGoey 2007). Nurses over many years have experienced how non-nurses use obtuseness (Sedgwick 2008) to not hear, listen or see what nurses reveal. Nursing's long-standing efforts devoted over the years to proving how essential it is to safe and effective healthcare is a striking example of this powerful form of ignorance. What would happen if we spent time working on knowledge important to nurses and nursing? The kind of scholarship taken up here, from a variety of disciplines, should therefore be valued, and broader discussions about them should take place in nursing and healthcare. Importantly, such issues must be discussed with students, but not as problems that can be addressed through research, science, or even bioethics, which, in our view, cannot engage with the politics of healthcare, nursing and everyday life. Feminist and postcolonial epistemologies and ethics, for example, provide a much more fertile ground to engage with issues of subjectivities, embodiment, the connectedness of the subject and the world, knowledge and power transactions—and ignorance.

Uncertainty and multiple other forms of unknown are prevalent in nursing; they emerge from epistemic privilege, a form of active ignorance that prevents one from recognising 'the intelligibility and validity of [another person's] perspective' (Medina 2011: 28). In such instances, ignorance is mobilised to discredit (an)other's thoughts, actions or sentiments, resulting in an inability to understand and respond to a situation. While this mobilisation signals an abuse of ignorance in nursing, it speaks to why nurses feel they are not heard in the healthcare system. Yet, as Townley (2006, 2011) and other feminists assert (e.g. Code 2004; Sullivan and Tuana 2007), ignorance can be mobilised to suspend assumptions of knowing, when we recognise that we are ill-equipped to know (Medina 2011). Code asserts that there is no space free of ignorance, pointing to 'the impotence of the epistemologies of mastery'

(Code 2004: 299), particularly in answering the challenges that confront us in healthcare.

One preliminary aspect of a solution may rest in what Funtowicz and Ravetz (1993: 753) call *postnormal science*—a kind of science where 'local, personal knowledge [and] extended facts' are brought into scientific debates in which science's putative 'veil of neutrality' can be challenged (Code 2013: 842). Science would no longer be the exclusive purview of scientists, but that of a broader, more inclusive community of peers who live with the consequences of production and integration of science in public policy. For these authors, postnormal science promotes dialogue with other realms of knowing grounded in ethics, spirituality, embodiment of experiences, and confessions to political commitments. In our view, this is so because postnormal science can recognise the inescapable fact that science interacts with the social. Such interactions already exist (Hulme 2007) and, despite scientists' best efforts to control bias and other 'polluting' influences, we need to stop pretending that social–science transactions have no bearing on knowledge—that values, beliefs and judgments do not pre-emptively influence experimental research, that they have no bearing on the formulation of research questions, the selection of study variables and endpoints, the design of experiments or statistical analyses, or the decisions about which findings get published and which do not (Smith 2005). Because ignorance is not properly addressed or valued as something worthy of inquiry, scientific traditions and education have fostered 'ignorance of ignorance', the attitude and accompanying practices that cast ignorance as something that can simply be ignored (Ravetz 1993) because it does not align easily with long-standing epistemological commitments. A postnormal reading of knowledge and scientific inquiry may accommodate insightful discussions about ignorance as a productive feature of the social because it deconstructs the epistemology of mastery that informs current scientific practices and, among other things, positions the unknown as a problem in the realm of knowledge production, rather than outside its calculations. In doing so, it makes room for local, uncoded ways of knowing that reflect temporal and spatial contingencies and that are responsive to day-to-day life and practices.

As members of a ramifying, heterogeneous epistemic community, nurses can partake in this endeavour by engaging openly and forcefully with the generative capacities of ignorance. They can thus tackle the blind spots, the uncertainties, the dangerous knowledges within their practice; practices such as deceit, denial and (racial, gender, etc.) discrimination; and unsettling states such as disgust and abjection. They can also interrogate the various ways in which nurses (and patients) are construed as risk (clinical, organisational, epistemic)—a liability to the smooth operations of clinical and administrative processes if they do not fully endorse, comply with and perpetuate managerialist thinking and solutions, which are characteristically geared toward control of nurses' work rather than their 'professional development'. By engaging with peers in such epistemic communities, nurses can question, problematise and resist the ways in which they themselves, and patients, are assigned non-knowing positions, subjected to external knowledge imposed top-down, and made responsible for systemic failures. As Townley argues:

> I need membership in a community of epistemic agents who will advise and correct me as I cultivate, refine, and maintain skills of reasoning and inquiry... People's epistemic agency can be limited if others refuse to acknowledge it—if they are discredited, dismissed, excluded, or treated merely instrumentally. Even if an agent's capacity to collect information remains intact under such conditions of epistemic injustice, her epistemic agency is impaired when she is denied full membership in the broader epistemic community... [We] need to take seriously matters of social position, race, gender, sexuality, and the like because social hierarchies can both limit the spheres of action available to agents from non-privileged groups and discourage those from privileged groups from being accountable for their actions when they seek and claim knowledge.
>
> Townley (2006: 40)

Nurses can remain highly sceptical of tools and solutions that only postpone the difficult realisation that these issues are pervasive, that they have not gone, and will not go, away. A decision not to engage with these uncomfortable questions may be grounded in ignorance of their existence or import, but it can also constitute a flight strategy to escape confronting discussions and uncomfortable states. But flight only breeds more ignorance. If we recognise that ignorance is ever-present, then acknowledgement of what one does not know affords nurses a place for response-ability (Latimer and Munro, 2015) that does not follow paths and guidelines set within managerialism, but allows trust to be built around what is acknowledged as mutually unknown (Townley 2006). Calls to mastery ascribed by expertise can be resisted. Instead, we propose an ethics of discomfort leading to empathic positioning through self-awareness and response-ability. To achieve this, we need to learn to be comfortable with discomfort (Perron et al. 2014) and teach students the same, as a step toward epistemic justice. Mastery is unlikely; instead we should, as Socrates suggested, move from the first premise of ignorance. Townley (2006) suggests that taking such an epistemic position affords a point of view of 'knowing this much' while also recognising that 'I do not know'—I am ignorant from your perspective. As Medina (2011) emphasises, such use of ignorance affords a position of epistemic justice rather than privilege, where ignorance, rather than preventing recognition of the intelligibility and validity of a person's point of view, allows the suspension of knowledge. This will lead nurses to be positioned in a zone of discomfort (Perron et al. 2014) in recognition of their incomplete knowledge, thereby positioning them as empathically—and knowingly— ignorant.

Abbreviations

BPG	best practice guideline
EBM	evidence-based medicine
EBMWG	Evidence-Based Medicine Working Group
EBN	evidence-based nursing
EBP	evidence-based practice
ePD	emancipatory practice development
GISRS	Global Influenza Surveillance and Response System
JBI	Joanna Briggs Institute
KU	knowledge utilisation
RCT	randomised controlled trial
WHO	World Health Organization

References

AACN (2014). 'Clinical habits die hard: Nursing traditions often trump evidence-based practice.' *ScienceDaily* April 1. [Online], Available: www.sciencedaily.com/releases/2014/04/140401101847.htm [accessed 9 July 2014].

Ahern, K. and S. McDonald (2002). 'The beliefs of nurses who were involved in a whistleblowing event.' *Journal of Advanced Nursing* 38(3): 303–309.

Ahmed, S. (2008). 'The politics of good feeling.' *Australian Critical Race and Whiteness Studies Association e-Journal* 4(1): 1–18.

Alavi, C. (2005). 'Breaking-in bodies: teaching nursing, initiations, or What's love got to do with it?' *Contemporary Nurse* 18(3): 292–299.

Alcoff, L.M. (2007). 'Epistemologies of ignorance: Three types.' *Race and Epistemologies of Ignorance*. S. Sullivan and N. Tuana. Albany, NY, State University of New York Press: 39–58.

Alcoff, L. and E. Potter (1993). *Feminist Epistemologies*. New York, Routledge.

Allen, D. (1985). 'Nursing research and social control: alternative models of science that emphasize understanding and emancipation.' *Image: The Journal of Nursing Scholarship* 17(2): 58–64.

Allen, D. (2013). 'Editorial. The sociology of care work.' *Sociology of Health and Illness*. [Online], Available: http://onlinelibrary.wiley.com/journal/10.1111/%28ISSN%291467-9566/homepage/the_sociology_of_care.htm [accessed 18 February 2015].

Allen, D. (2015). *The Invisible Work of Nurses: Hospitals, Organisation and Healthcare*. Abingdon, UK, Routledge.

Allen, D., D. Hughes and R. Dingwall (2013). 'Introduction: The Francis reports: Care standards, regulation and accountability.' *Sociology of Health and Illness*. [Online], Available: http://onlinelibrary.wiley.com/journal/10.1111/%28ISSN%291467-9566/homepage/virtual_special_issue_series__the_francis_reports.htm [accessed 18 February 2015].

Alvesson, M. and A. Spicer (2012). 'A stupidity-based theory of organizations.' *Journal of Management Studies* 49: 1194–1220.

ANA (2010). 'ANA urges registered nurses to get the seasonal influenza vaccine.' American Nurses Association. [Online], Available: www.nursingworld.org/FunctionalMenuCategories/MediaResources/PressReleases/2010-PR/ANA-Urges-RNs-Get-Seasonal-Influenza-Vaccine.pdf [accessed 23 August 2014].

Anema, M.G. and J. McCoy (2010). *Competency-Based Nursing Education. Guide to Achieving Outstanding Learner Outcomes*. New York, Springer.

Andrews, G.J. and R. Kitchin (2005). 'Geography and nursing: Convergence in cyberspace.' *Nursing Inquiry* 12(4): 316–324.

Anonymous (1996). 'News: Breaking the impotence taboo.' *Journal of Advanced Nursing* 24: 428.

Armstrong, R. (2015). Ruth Armstrong: Battlelines, 9 February. [Online], Available: www.mja.com.au/insight/2015/4/ruth-armstrong-battlelines.

Attard, M. (2009). 'Carriers of responsibility: an existential encounter with parents who know their child is, or could be, a carrier of a mutation in the cystic fibrosis gene.' PhD thesis, Sydney Nursing School, University of Sydney.

Bail, K., R. Cook, A. Gardner and L. Grealish (2009). 'Writing ourselves into a web of obedience: a nursing policy analysis.' *International Journal of Nursing Studies* 46: 1457–1466.

Bailey, A. (2007). 'Strategic ignorance.' *Race and Epistemologies of Ignorance*. S. Sullivan and N. Tuana. Albany, NY, State University of New York Press: 77–92.

Ballard, T., C. Davie, W. Offley, J. Tino, C. Vanderbyl, T. Visser et al. Influenza vaccination (June 2013). [Online], Available: www.canadian-nurse.com/articles/issues/2013/june-2013/influenza-vaccination [accessed 10 February 2015].

Barbee, E.L. (1993). 'Racism in US nursing.' *Medical Anthropology Quarterly New Series, Racism, Gender, Class and Health* 7(4): 346–362.

Barnes, L. and T. Rudge (2005). 'Virtual reality or real virtuality: the space of flows and nursing practice.' *Nursing Inquiry* 12(4): 306–315.

Barnum, B.J.S. (1998). *Nursing Theory: Analysis, Application, Evaluation* (5th edn). Philadelphia, PA, J. B. Lippincott.

Basford, L. and O. Slevin (2003). *Theory and Practice of Nursing: An Integrated Approach to Caring Practice* (2nd edn). Cheltenham, UK, Nelson Thornes.

Bauman, Z. (2000). *Liquid Modernity*. Cambridge, Polity.

Bauman, Z. (2001). *The Individualized Society*. Cambridge, Polity.

Bauman, Z. (2004). *Wasted Lives: Modernity and its Outcasts*. Oxford, Polity.

Bauman, Z. (2011). *Collateral Damage: Social Inequalities in a Global Age*. Cambridge, Polity.

Baumann, A.O., R.B. Deber and G.G. Thompson (1991). 'Overconfidence among physicians and nurses: the "micro-certainty, macro-uncertainty" phenomenon.' *Social Science and Medicine* 32(2): 167–174.

BCCDC (2013). *BC Influenza Prevention Policy: A Discussion of the Evidence*. Vancouver, British Columbia Centre for Disease Control.

Beardwood, B.A. and J.M. Kainer (2013). 'Exploring risk in professional nursing practice: an analysis of work refusal and professional risk.' *Nursing Inquiry* 2013: 1–13.

Beck, U. (1992). *Risk Society: Towards a New Modernity*. New Delhi, Sage.

Beck, U. (1995). *Ecological Enlightenment : Essays on the Politics of the Risk Society*. Atlantic Highlands, NJ,Humanities Press.

Beck, U. (2000). 'Risk society revisited: Theory, politics, and research programmes.' *The Risk Society and Beyond. Critical Issues for Social Theory*. B. Adam, U. Beck and J. Van Loon. Thousand Oaks, CA, Sage: 211–229.

Beck, U. and B. Holzer (2007). 'Organizations in world risk society.' *International Handbook of Organizational Crisis Management*. C. Pearson, C. Roux-Dufort and J. Clair. Thousand Oaks, CA, Sage: 3–25.

Benedict, S. and L. Shields (2014). *Nurses and Midwives in Nazi Germany: The 'Euthanasia Programs*. New York, Routledge [ebook].

Benjamin, M. and J. Curtis (2010). *Ethics in Nursing: Cases, Principles, and Reasoning* (3rd edn). New York, Oxford University Press.

Benner, P., C.Tanner and C. Chesla (2009). *Expertise in Nursing Practice, Second Edition: Caring, Clinical Judgment, and Ethics.* New York, Springer.

Berragan, L. (1998). 'Nursing practice draws upon several different ways of knowing.' *Journal of Clinical Nursing* 7: 209–217.

Bilton, R. (2014). 'Apple "failing to protect Chinese factory workers".' BBC December 18. [Online], Available: www.bbc.com/news/business-30532463 [accessed 6 January 2015].

Binns, T. (2007). 'Marginal lands, marginal geographies.' *Progress in Human Geography* 31(5): 587–591.

Bjerg, K. (1967). 'The suicidal life spaces: Attempts at a reconstruction from suicide notes.' *Essays in Self Destruction.* E.S. Shneidman. New York, Science House: 475–493.

Blakemore, S. (2009). 'How productive wards can improve patient care.' *Nursing Management* 16(5): 14–18.

Bok, S. (1983). 'The limits of confidentiality.' *The Hastings Center Report* 13(1): 24–31.

Bok, S. (1989). *Secrets. On the Ethics of Concealment and Revelation.* New York, Vintage Books.

Bourdieu, P. (1977). *Outline of a Theory of Practice.*Cambridge, Cambridge University Press.

Bourgeault, G. (1999). *Éloge de l'incertitude.* Montréal, Éditions Bellarmin.

Boyer, K. (2011). '"The way to break the taboo is to do the taboo thing": Breastfeeding in public and citizen-activism in the UK.' *Health & Place* 17: 430–437.

Braaten, J. (1990). 'Towards a feminist reassessment of intellectual virtue.' *Hypatia* 5: 1–14.

Bradbury-Jones, C. and J. Taylor (2014). 'Domestic abuse as transgressive practice: Understanding nurses' responses through the lens of abjection.' *Nursing Philosophy* 14: 295–304.

Brown, C. and J. Cataldo (2013). 'Exploration of lung cancer stigma for female long-term survivors.' *Nursing Inquiry* 20(4): 352–362.

Buchak, L. (2013). *Risk and Rationality.* Oxford, Oxford University Press.

Burke, J. (2013). 'Bangladesh factory collapse leaves trail of shattered lives.' *The Guardian* June 6. [Online], Available: www.theguardian.com/world/2013/jun/06/bangladesh-factory-building-collapse-community [accessed 6 January 2015].

Burnard, P. (1998). 'The last two taboos in community nursing.' *Journal of Community Nursing* 12(4): 4–6.

Burston, S., W. Chaboyer, M. Wallis, and J. Stanfield (2011). 'A discussion of approaches to transforming care: Contemporary strategies to improve patient safety.' *Journal of Advanced Nursing* 67(11): 2488–2495.

Butterworth, T. (2014). 'Board editorial: The nursing profession and its leaders – hiding in plain sight?' *Journal of Research in Nursing* 19(7/8): 533–536.

Canadian Task Force on the Periodic Health Examination (1979). 'Task Force Report. The Periodic Health Examination.' *Canadian Medical Association Journal* 121(9): 1193–1254.

Carolan, M., G.J. Andrews and E. Hodnett (2006). 'Writing place: a comparison of nursing research and health geography.' *Nursing Inquiry* 13(3): 201–219.

Carper, B.A. (1978). 'Fundamental patterns of knowing in nursing.' *Advances in Nursing Science* 1(1): 13–24.

Cartwright, N. (2007). 'Are RCTs the gold standard?' *BioSocieties* 2: 11–20.

CDC (2012). 'CDC recommendations for influenza antiviral medications remain unchanged.' Centers for Disease Control and Prevention, February 7. [Online],

Available: www.cdc.gov/media/haveyouheard/stories/Influenza_antiviral.html [accessed 29 December 2014].

Ceci, C. (2004). 'Gender, power, nursing: A case analysis.' *Nursing Inquiry* 11(2): 72–81.

CFNU (2012). 'CFNU position statement on mandatory influenza immunization. Mandatory influenza immunization of nurses: Unethical and unnecessary.' Canadian Federation of Nurses Unions. [Online], Available: https://nursesunions.ca/sites/default/files/postition_statement_mandatory_immunization.pdf [accessed 12 November 2014].

Chanter, T. (2006). 'Abjection and the constitutive nature of difference: class mourning in Margaret's museum and legitimating myths of innocence in Casablanca.' *Hypatia* 21(3): 86–106.

Charlton, B.G. and A. Miles (1998). 'The rise and fall of EBM.' *QJM – An International Journal of Medicine* 91(5): 371–374.

CNA (2012). Position Statement. Influenza immunization of registered nurses. Canadian Nurses Association. [Online], Available: https://www.cna-aiic.ca/~/media/cna/page-content/pdf-fr/ps_influenza_immunization_for_rns_e.pdf [accessed 23 August 2014].

Cochrane Collaboration and BMJ (2014). News Release. Tamiflu and Relenza: How effective are they? April 10. [Online], Available: www.cochrane.org/features/tamiflu-relenza-how-effective-are-they [accessed 9 January 2015].

Code, L. (1991). *What Can She Know?* Ithaca, NY, Cornell University Press.

Code, L. (2004). 'The power of ignorance.' *Philosophical Papers* 33(3): 291–308.

Code, L. (2008a). 'Advocacy, negotiation, and the politics of unknowing.' *Southern Journal of Philosophy* 46(S1): 32–51.

Code, L. (2008b). 'Thinking about ecological thinking.' *Hypatia* 23(1): 187–203.

Code, L. (2013). 'Doubt and denial: Epistemic responsibility meets climate change scepticism.' *Oñati Socio-Legal Series* 3(5): 838–853.

Code, L. (2014). 'Culpable ignorance?' *Hypatia* 29(3): 670–676.

Cohen, D. and P. Carter (2010). 'WHO and the pandemic flu "conspiracies".' *British Medical Journal* 340: c2912.

College and Association of Registered Nurses of Alberta (2014). 'Registered nurses first regulator to issue position statement on mandatory influenza immunization.' [Online], Available: www.nurses.ab.ca/content/carna/home/current-issues-and-events/media-resources/media-release-2/oct-6-2014.html [accessed 12 December 2014].

Connell, E. and A. Hunt (2010). 'The HPV Vaccination Campaign: A project of moral regulation in an era of biopolitics.' *Canadian Journal of Sociology/Cahiers canadiens de sociologie* 35(1): 63–82.

Conner, C.D. (2005). *A People's History of Science: Miners, Midwives, and "Low Mechanics"*. New York, Nation Books.

Cook, C. (2009). 'Women's health theorizing: a call for epistemic action.' *Critical Public Health* 19(2):143–154.

Croissant, J.L. (2014). 'Agnatology: Ignorance and absence or towards a sociology of things that aren't there.' *Social Epistemology* 28(1): 4–25.

Curley, S.P., S.A. Eraker and J.F. Yates (1984). 'An investigation of patients' reactions to therapeutic uncertainty.' *Medical Decision Making* 4(4): 501–511.

D'Antonio, P. (2006). 'History for a practice profession.' *Nursing Inquiry* 13(4): 242–248.

Davies, W. and L. McGoey (2014). 'Rationalities of ignorance: on financial crisis and the ambivalence of neo-liberal epistemology.' *Economy and Society* 41(1): 64–83.

Davis, M., P. Flowers and N. Stephenson (2013). '"We had to do what we thought was right at the time": Retrospective discourse on the 2009 H1N1 pandemic in the UK.' *Sociology of Health and Illness* 36(3): 369–382.

De Koninck, T. (2000). *La nouvelle ignorance et le problème de la culture.* Vendôme, Presses Universitaires de France.

Demicheli, V., T. Jefferson, A.L. Al-Ansary, E. Ferroni, A. Rivetti and C. Di Pietrantonj (2014). 'Vaccines for preventing influenza in healthy adults.' *Cochrane Database of Systematic Reviews* 2014(3): CD001269. DOI: 10.1002/14651858.CD001269.pub5.

Dodge, M. and R. Kitchin (2013). 'Crowdsourced cartography: Mapping experience and knowledge.' *Environment and Planning A* 45: 19–36.

Donaldson, S.K. and D.M. Crowley (1978). 'The discipline of nursing.' *Nursing Outlook* 26(2): 113–120.

Douglas, M. (1992). *Risk and Blame: Essays in Cultural Theory.* London, Routledge.

Douglas, M. (2002). *Purity and Danger.* London, Routledge.

Dreyfus, H. and P. Rabinow (1982). *Michel Foucault: Beyond Structuralism and Hermeneutics.* Chicago, IL, Chicago University Press.

Duff, C. (2010). 'On the role of affect and practice in the production of place.' *Environment and Planning D: Society and Space* 28: 881–895.

Duncan, R. and M. Weston-Smith (1984). *The Encyclopaedia of Medical Ignorance: Exploring the Frontiers of Medical Knowledge.* Elsmford, NY, Pergamon Press.

Dunn, A.G., D. Arachi, J. Hudgins, G. Tsafnat, E. Coiera and F. Bourgeois (2014). 'Financial conflicts of interest and conclusions about neuraminidase inhibitors for influenza: An analysis of systematic reviews.' *Annals of Internal Medicine* 161(7): 513–518.

Ehrich, K.R. and J.R. Irwin (2005). 'Willful ignorance in the request for product attribute information.' *Journal of Marketing Research,*42(3): 266–277.

Ellis, P. (2014). *Understanding Ethics for Nursing Students.* London, Learning Matters.

Estabrooks, C.A., L. Dersken, C. Winther, J.N. Lavis, S.D. Scott, L.Wallin and J. Profetto-McGrath (2008). 'The intellectual structure and substance of the knowledge utilization field: a longitudinal author co-citation analysis, 1945 to 2004.' *Implementation Science* 3: 49–70.

Evans, A. (2010). 'Strange yet compelling: Anxiety and abjection in hospital nursing.' *Abjectly Boundless: Boundaries, Bodies and Health Work.* T. Rudge and D. Holmes. Farnham, UK: Ashgate: 191–211.

Every-Palmer, S. and J. Howick (2014). 'How evidence-based medicine is failing due to biased trials and selective publication.' *Journal of Evaluation in Clinical Practice* 20(6): 908–914.

Faulkner, A. (1985). 'The consequences of ignorance: Nurse–patient communication.' *Consensus and Penalties for Ignorance in the Medical Sciences: Implications for Information Transfer* (British Library research report). M.J. Brittain. London, Taylor Graham: 121–135.

Feenan, D. (2007) 'Understanding disadvantage partly through an epistemology of ignorance.' *Social and Legal Studies* 16(4): 509–531.

Firestein, S. (2012). *Ignorance: How it Drives Science.* New York, Oxford University Press.

Foth, T. (2009). 'Biopolitical spaces, vanished death, and the power of vulnerability in nursing.' *Aporia* 1(4): 16–26.

Foucault, M. (1970). *The Order of Things.* London, Tavistock.

Foucault, M. (1977). *Discipline and Punish: The Birth of the Prison.* London, Tavistock.

Foucault, M. (1978). *History of Sexuality, Vol. 1. The Will to Knowledge.* London, Penguin.

Foucault, M. (1991) 'Governmentality.' *The Foucault Effect. Studies in Governmentality.* G. Burchell, C. Gordon and P. Miller. Chicago, IL, Chicago University Press: 87–104.

Foucault, M. (2007). *Security, Territory, Population: Lectures at the College de France 1977–78.*New York, Palgrave Macmillan.

Francis, R. (2010) *Independent Inquiry into care provided by Mid Staffordshire NHS Foundation Trust January 2005–March 2009.* London, The Stationery Office. http://webarchive.nationalarchives.gov.uk/20130107105354/http://www.dh.gov.uk/en/Publicationsandstatistics/Publications/PublicationsPolicyAndGuidance/DH_113018

Francis, R. (2013) *Report of the Mid Staffordshire NHS Foundation Trust Public Inquiry.* London, The Stationery Office. www.midstaffspublicinquiry.com/report

Freeman, M. and P. Jaoudé (2007). 'Justifying surgery's last taboo: The ethics of face transplants.' *Journal of Medical Ethics* 33: 76–81.

French, B. (2002). 'Uncertainty and information need in nursing.' *Nurse Education Today* 26: 245–252.

Freshwater, D. (2004). 'Globalisation and innovation: Nursing's role in creating a participative knowledge economy.' *Nursing Times Research* 9(4): 240–242.

Freud, S. (1955/1985). *Totem and Taboo: Some Points of Agreement between the Mental Lives of Savages and Neurotics.* The Pelican Freud Library, Volume 13. Harmondsworth, UK, Penguin.

Frickel, S., S. Gibbon, J. Howard, J. Kempner, G. Ottinger and D.J. Hess (2010). 'Undone science: Charting social movement and civil society challenges to research agenda setting.' *Science, Technology, and Human Values* 35(4): 444–473.

Funtowicz, S. and J. Ravetz (1993). 'Science for the post-normal age.' *Futures* 25(7): 739–755.

Gagnon, M. (2010). 'Managing the other within the self: Bodily experiences of HIV/AIDS.' *Abjectly Boundless: Boundaries, Bodies and Health Work.* T. Rudge and D. Holmes. Farnham, UK, Ashgate: 133–145.

Gammage, W. (2012). *The Greatest Estate on Earth.* Sydney, Allen and Unwin.

Garfinkel, H. (1967). 'Practical sociological reasoning: Some features in the work of the Los Angeles Suicide Prevention Centre.' *Essays in Self Destruction.* E.S. Shneidman. New York, Science House: 171–187.

Garling, P. (2008). *Final Report of the Special Commission of Inquiry: Acute Care Services in NSW Public Hospitals.* Sydney, State of NSW. [Online], Available: http://www.dpc.nsw.gov.au/__data/assets/pdf_file/0003/34194/Overview_-_Special_Commission_Of_Inquiry_Into_Acute_Care_Services_In_New_South_Wales_Public_Hospitals.pdf [accessed July 2015].

Gaudet, J. (2013). 'It takes two to tango: Knowledge mobilization and ignorance mobilization in science research and innovation.' *Prometheus: Critical Studies in Innovation* 31(3): 169–187.

Gaudet, J., N. Young and M. Gross (2012). *Ignorance is Power.* Canadian Sociological Association Conference, Kitchener-Waterloo, Canada.

Gaztambide-Ferdandez, R. (2012). 'Editorial: Our passion for ignorance.' *Curriculum Inquiry* 42(4): 445–453.

Gibbs, L. and E. Gambrill (2002). 'Evidence-based practice: Counterarguments to objections.' *Research on Social Work Practice* 12(3): 452–476.

Giddens, A. (1991). *Modernity and Self-Identity. Self and Society in the Late Modern Age.* Stanford, CA, Stanford University Press.

Giddens, A. (1999). 'Risk and responsibility.' *Modern Law Review* 62(1): 1–10.

Ginzburg, C. (1989). *Clues, Myths, and the Historical Method.* Trans. J. Tedeschi and A. Tedeschi. Baltimore, MD, Johns Hopkins University Press.

Giroux, H. (2014). *The Violence of Organized Forgetting: Thinking beyond America's Disimagination Machine*. San Francisco, CA, City Lights Books.

Glen, S. (1997). 'Confidentiality: A critique of the traditional view.' *Nursing Ethics* 4(5): 403–406.

Gluyas, H., S. Alliex and P. Morrison (2011). 'Do enquiries into health system failures lead to change in clinical governance?' *Collegian* 18: 147–155.

Goffman, E. (1968). *Stigma: Notes on the Management of Spoiled Identity*. Harmondsworth, UK, Penguin.

Goffman, E. (1969). *Presentation of Self in Everyday Life*. New York, Doubleday.

Goldacre, B. (2006). 'Archie Cochrane: "Fascist".' August 19. [Online], Available: www.badscience.net/2006/08/archie-cochrane-fascist/ [accessed 12 September 2014].

Goldenberg, M.J. (2009). 'Iconoclast or creed? Objectivism, pragmatism and the hierarchy of evidence.' *Perspectives in Biology and Medicine* 52(2): 168–187.

Gordon, S. (2002). 'Thinking like a nurse: You have to be a nurse to do it.' *Nursing Inquiry* 9(1): 57–61.

Graham, I.D., J. Logan, M.B. Harrison, S.E. Straus, J. Tetroe, W. Caswell and N. Robinson (2006). 'Lost in knowledge translation: Time for a map?' *Journal of Continuing Education in the Health Professions* 26(1): 13–24.

Greer, G. (2004). 'Whitefella jump up: Response to correspondence.' *Quarterly Essay* 14: 109–116.

Gross, M. (2007). 'The unknown in process: dynamic connections of ignorance, non-knowledge and related concepts.' *Current Sociology* 55(5): 742–759.

Grove, W.M., D.H. Zald, B.S. Lebow, B.E. Snitz and C. Nelson (2000). 'Clinical versus mechanical prediction: A meta-analysis.' *Psychological Assessment* 12(1): 19–30.

Haaretz (2015). 'Thai workers in Israel suffer serious labor abuse, rights group says.' *Haaretz* January 25. [Online], Available: www.haaretz.com/news/national/1.638779 [6 Jan 2015].

Haebich, A. (2011). 'Forgetting Indigenous histories: Cases from the history of Australia's stolen generations.' *Journal of Social History* 44(4): 1033–1046.

Hage, G. (1998). *White Nation: Fantasies of White Supremacy in a Multicultural Society*. Annandale, NSW, Pluto Press.

Halls v. Mitchell, Supreme Court of Canada (1928). S.C.R. 125. [Online], Available: http://scc-csc.lexum.com/scc-csc/scc-csc/en/item/3427/index.do [accessed 28 January 2015].

Hancock, K., J.M. Clayton, S.M. Parker et al. (2007). 'Truth-telling in discussing prognosis in advanced life-limiting illnesses: A systematic review.' *Palliative Medicine* 21: 507–517.

Haraway, D. (1989). 'The biopolitics of postmodern bodies: Determination of self in immune system discourse.' *Differences: A Journal of Feminist Cultural Studies* 1(1): 3–43.

Harding, S. (2006). 'Two influential theories of ignorance and philosophy's interests in ignoring them.' *Hypatia* 21(3): 20–36.

Harris, O. (1995). '"The coming of the white people": Reflections on the mythologisation of history in Latin America.' *Bulletin of Latin American Research* (special issue: Shifting Frontiers: Historical transformations of identities in Latin America) 14(1): 9–24.

Harrison, P. (2000). 'Making sense: embodiment and sensibilities of the everyday.' *Environment and Planning D: Society and Space* 18: 497–517.

Harvey, K. and T. Faunce (2006). 'A critical analysis of overseas-trained doctor ("OTD") factors in the Bundaberg Base Hospital Surgical Inquiry.' *Law in Context* 23(2): 73–90.

Heartfield, M. (2002). 'Governing recovery: A discourse analysis of hospital length of stay.' PhD thesis, University of Melbourne, Australia.

Hoagland, S.L. (2007). 'Denying relationality: Epistemology and ethics and ignorance.' *Race and Epistemologies of Ignorance*. S. Sullivan and N. Tuana. Albany, NY, SUNY Press: 95–118.

Holmes, D. and C. Federman (2003). 'Killing for the state: the darkest side of American nursing.' *Nursing Inquiry* 10(1): 2–10.

Holmes, D. and C. Federman. (2010). 'Fearing sex: Toxic bodies, paranoia and the rise of technophilia.' *Abjectly Boundless: Boundaries, Bodies and Health Work*. T. Rudge and D. Holmes. Farnham, UK: Ashgate: 67–80.

Holmes, D. and D. Gastaldo (2002). 'Nursing as means of governmentality.' *Journal of Advanced Nursing* 38: 557–565.

Holmes, D., S. Murray, A. Perron and G. Rail (2006a). 'Deconstructing the evidence-based discourse in health sciences: Truth, power, and fascism.' *International Journal of Evidence Based Health Care* 4: 180–186.

Holmes, D., A. Perron and P. O'Byrne (2006b). 'Understanding disgust in nursing: Abjection, self and the other.' *Research and Theory for Nursing Practice: An International Journal* 20(4): 305–315.

Hope, T. (1995). 'Deception and lying.' *Journal of Medical Ethics* 21(2): 67–68.

Houppert, K. (1999). *The Curse: Confronting the Last Unmentionable Taboo: Menstruation*. New York, Farrar, Straus and Giroux.

Hughes, D. (2013). *Sociological Perspectives on Regulation and Governance: The Francis Reports*. Virtual Special Issue Series, Sociology of Health & Illness. Oxford, Wiley.

Hulme, M. (2007). 'The appliance of science.' *The Guardian* March 14. [Online], Available: www.theguardian.com/society/2007/mar/14/scienceofclimatechange.climatechange [accessed 21 July 2014].

Hume, S. (1994). 'History's march over ignorance.' *The Vancouver Sun* 12 January, A11.

ICN (2013). *Fact Sheet. Immunisations for Health-care Workers: Influenza and Hepatitis B*. Geneva, International Council of Nurses. [Online], Available: www.icn.ch/images/stories/documents/publications/fact_sheets/4d_FS-Immunisations_HC_workers.pdf [accessed 2 February 2015].

Institute of Medicine (2010). *The Future of Nursing: Leading Change, Advancing Health*. Washington, DC, National Academies Press.

Jefferson, T., A. Rivetti, A. Harnden, C. Di Pietrantonj and V. Demicheli (2008). 'Vaccines for preventing influenza in healthy children.' *Cochrane Database of Systematic Reviews* 2008(2): CD004879. DOI: 10.1002/14651858.CD004879.pub3.

Jefferson, T., C. Di Pietrantonj, L.A. Al-Ansary, E. Ferroni, S. Thorning and R.E. Thomas (2010a). 'Vaccines for preventing influenza in the elderly.' *Cochrane Database of Systematic Reviews* 2010(2): CD004876. DOI: 10.1002/14651858.

Jefferson, T., C. Di Pietrantonj, A. Rivetti, G.A. Bawazeer, L.A. Al-Ansary and E. Ferroni (2010b). 'Vaccines for preventing influenza in healthy adults.' *Cochrane Database of Systematic Reviews* 2010(7): CD001269. DOI: 10.1002/14651858.CD001269.pub4.

Jefferson, T., M. Jones, P. Doshi, E.A. Spencer, I. Onakpoya and C.J. Heneghan (2014a). 'Oseltamivir for influenza in adults and children: systematic review of clinical study reports and summary of regulatory comments.' *British Medical Journal* 348: g2545. DOI: 10.1136/bmj.g2545.

Jefferson, T., M. Jones, P. Doshi, C.B. Del Mar, R. Hafma, M.J. Thompson et al. (2014b). 'Neuraminidase inhibitors for preventing and treating influenza in healthy adults and children.' *Cochrane Database of Systematic Reviews* 2014(4): CD008965. DOI: 10.1002/14651858.CD008965.pub4.

Jensen, K. (2014). 'Signing communities dealing with non-knowledge: Some cases from nursing.' *Professions and Professionalism* [Online], Available: https://journals. hioa.no/index.php/pp/article/view/824/816 [accessed 18 December 2014].

Jiménez-Jorge, S., S. de Mateo, C. Delgado-Sanz, F. Pozo, I. Casas, M. Garcia-Cenoz et al. (2013). 'Effectiveness of influenza vaccine against laboratory-confirmed influenza, in the late 2011–2012 season in Spain, among population targeted for vaccination.' *BMC Infectious Diseases* 13: 441–453. DOI: 10.1186/1471-2334-13-441.

Johnson, M. (1999). 'Observations on positivism and pseudoscience in qualitative nursing research.' *Journal of Advanced Nursing* 30: 67–73.

Johnstone, M.-J. (2011) *Bioethics: A Nursing Perspective*, 5th edn. Chatswood, NSW, Elsevier.

Jones, D. (2012). 'History and ignorance are bad bedfellows.' *Evening Standard, London*, 2 July: 15.

Jutel, A. (2008). 'Beyond evidence-based nursing: tools for practice.' *Journal of Nursing Management* 16: 417–421.

Kagan, P.N., M.C. Smith and P.L. Chinn (2014). *Philosophies and Practices of Emancipatory Nursing: Social Justice as Praxis*. New York, Routledge.

Keighley, T. (2012). 'Globalization, decision making and taboo in nursing.' *International Nursing Review* 59: 181–186.

Keller, J.G. and D.B. Keller (2011). 'Socrates, dialogue, and us: ignorance as learning paradigm.' *Epistemologies of Ignorance in Education*. E. Malewski and N. Jaramillo. Charlotte, NC, Information Age Publishers: 87–104.

Kempner, J., J. Merz and C. Bosk (2011). 'Forbidden knowledge: Public controversy and the production of non-knowledge.' *Sociological Forum* 26(3): 475–500.

Kerwin, A. (1993). 'None to solid: medical ignorance.' *Science Communication* 15: 166–185.

Kipnis, A. (2008). 'Audit cultures: neoliberal governmentality, socialist legacy, or technologies of governing.' *American Ethnologist* 35(2): 275–289.

Kleinman, D. and S. Suryanarayanan (2012). 'Dying bees and the social production of ignorance.' *Science, Technology, and Human Values* 38(4): 492–517.

Knaapen, L. (2013). 'Being "evidence-based" in the absence of evidence: The management of non-evidence in guideline development.' *Social Studies of Science* 43(5): 681–706.

Kristeva, J. (1982). *Powers of Horror: An Essay on Abjection*. New York, Columbia University Press.

Kuznets, S. (1968). *Toward a Theory of Economic Growth*. New York, W.W. Norton and Co.

Lamont, L. (1997). 'Ignorance of history "risks crisis"'. *Sydney Morning Herald* [Late Edition]. 22 September: 3.

Lamont, P. and C. Bates (2007). 'Conjuring images of India in the nineteenth-century Britain.' *Social History* 32(3): 308–324

The Lamp (2006). 'Dr Death scandal reveals flawed system.' *The Lamp* 63: 33. [Online], Available: http://search.informit.com.au/documentSummary;dn=2044776 33800652;res=IELHEA [accessed 17 February 2015].

Landzelius, M. (2009). 'Spatial reification, or, collectively embodied amnesia, aphasia, and apraxia.' *Semiotician* 175(1/4): 39–75.

Latimer, J. (1999). 'The dark at the bottom of the stairs.' *Medical Anthropology Quarterly* 13(2): 186–213.

Latimer, J. (2010). 'Defacing horror, realigning nurses.' *Abjectly Boundless: Boundaries, Bodies and Health Work*. T. Rudge and D. Holmes. Farnham, UK, Ashgate: 265–274.

Latimer, J. (2014). 'Guest editorial: Nursing, the politics of organisation and meanings of care.' *Journal of Research in Nursing* 19(7/8): 537–545.

Latimer, J. and R. Munro (2015) 'Uprooting class? Culture, world-making and reform.' *Sociological Review* 63(2): 415–432.

Latour, B. (2004). *Politics of Nature: How to Bring the Sciences into Democracy*. Cambridge, MA, Harvard University Press.

Lau, D., J. Hu, S.R. Majumdar, D.A. Storie, S.E. Rees and J.A. Johnson (2012). 'Interventions to improve influenza and pneumococcal vaccination rates among community-dwelling adults: A systematic review and meta-analysis.' *Annals of Family Medicine* 10: 538–546.

Lawler, J. (1991). *Behind the Screens: Nursing, Somology and the Problem of the Body*. Melbourne, Churchill Livingstone.

Lawler, J. (Ed.) (2002). *The Body in Nursing: A Collection of Views*. Melbourne, Churchill Livingstone.

Lawton, J. (1998). 'Contemporary hospice care: The sequestration of the unbounded body.' *Sociology of Health and Illness* 20(2): 121–143.

Lehtinen, E. (2005). 'Information, understanding and the benign order of everyday life in genetic counselling.' *Sociology of Health and Illness* 27(5): 575–601.

Lemke, T. (2011). *Biopolitics. An Advanced Introduction*. New York, New York University Press.

Lenzer, J. (2015). 'Why aren't the US Centers for Disease Control and Food and Drug Administration speaking with one voice on flu?' *British Medical Journal* 350: h658. [Online], Available: www.bmj.com/content/350/bmj.h658 [accessed 6 February 2015].

Lewis, M.W. (2000). 'Global ignorance.' *Geographical Review* 90(4): 603–628.

Lindsay, B. (2004). 'Randomized controlled trials of socially complex nursing interventions: creating bias and unreliability.' *Journal of Advanced Nursing* 45(1): 84–94.

Locsin, R.C. and M.J. Purnell (2009). *A Contemporary Nursing Process: The (Un) Bearable Weight of Knowing in Nursing*. New York, Springer.

Lundvall, B.Å. and B. Johnson (1994). 'The learning economy.' *Journal of Industry Studies* 1(2): 23–42.

Lupton, D. (1999). *Risk*. London, Routledge.

Makic, M.B.F., C. Rauen, R. Watson and A.W. Poteet (2014). 'Examining the evidence to guide practice: Challenging practice habits.' *Critical Care Nurse* 34(2): 28–45.

Magnússon, S.G. (2010). *Wasteland with Words: A Social History of Iceland*. London, Reaktion Books.

Mair, J., A.H. Kelly and C. High, (2012). 'Introduction: Making ignorance an ethnographic object.' *The Anthropology of Ignorance: An Ethnographic Approach*. C. High, A.H. Kelly and J. Mari. New York, Palgrave Macmillan: 1–32.

Malewski, E. and N. Jaramillo (2011). 'Introduction.' *Epistemologies of Ignorance in Education*. E. Malewski and N. Jaramillo. Charlotte, NC, Information Age Publishers: 1–30.

Mansnerus, E. (2014). *Modelling in Public Health Research: How Mathematical Techniques Keep Us Healthy*. London, Palgrave Macmillan.

Masters, K. (2014). *Role Development in Professional Nursing Practice* (3rd edn). Burlington, MA, Jones and Bartlett Learning.

Mayor, A. (2008). 'Suppression of indigenous fossil knowledge: From Claverack, New York, 1705 to Agate Springs, Nebraska, 2005.' *Agnotology: The Making and*

Unmaking of Ignorance. R.N. Proctor and L. Schiebinger. Stanford, CA, Stanford University Press: 163–182

McCabe, J. (2010). 'Subjectivity and embodiment: Acknowledging abjection in nursing.' *Abjectly Boundless: Boundaries, Bodies, and Health Work*. T. Rudge and D. Holmes. Farnham, UK, Ashgate: 213–226.

McCarthy, M. (2014). 'Conflicts of interest may affect conclusions of systematic reviews of flu drugs, study indicates.' *British Medical Journal* 349: g6065.

McGeer, A. (2013). 'The risky business of influenza.' *Canadian Nurse* April. [Online], Available: www.canadian-nurse.com/articles/issues/2013/april-2013/the-risky-business-of-influenza [accessed 10 February 2015].

McGoey, L. (2007). 'On the will to ignorance in bureaucracy.' *Economy and Society* 36 (2): 212–235.

McGoey, L. (2012a). 'Strategic unknowns: towards a sociology of ignorance.' *Economy and Society* 41(1): 1–16.

McGoey, L. (2012b). 'The logic of strategic ignorance.' *British Journal of Sociology* 63(3): 553–576.

McKillop, A., N. Sheridan and D. Rowe (2013). 'New light through old windows: nurses, colonists and indigenous survival.' *Nursing Inquiry* 20(3): 265–276.

McLaren, P. (2011). 'Preface: Towards a decolonizing epistemology.'*Epistemologies of Ignorance in Education*. E. Malewski and N. Jaramillo. Charlotte, NC, Information Age Publishers: vii–xvii.

McMillan, I. (2008). 'Tackling taboos.' *Learning Disability Practice* 11(6): 3.

Medina, J. (2011). 'The relevance of credibility excess in a proportional view of epistemic injustice: differential epistemic authority and the social imaginary.' *Social Epistemology: A Journal of Knowledge, Culture and Policy* 25(1): 15–35.

Meleis, A.I. (2012). *Theoretical Nursing: Development and Progress* (5th edn). New York, Lippincott, Williams and Wilkins.

Meyer-Rochow, V. (2009). 'Food taboos: their origins and purposes.' *Journal of Ethnobiology and Ethnomedicine* 5: 18–27.

Michael, M. (1991). 'Discourses of danger and dangerous discourses: patrolling the borders of science, nature and society.' *Discourse and Society* 2(1), 5–28.

Miles, A., M. Loughlin, and A. Polychronis (2008). 'Evidence-based healthcare, clinical knowledge and the rise of personalised medicine.' *Journal of Evaluation in Clinical Practice* 14(5): 621–649.

Mills, C. (2007). 'White ignorance.' *Race and Epistemologies of Ignorance*. S. Sullivan and N. Tuana. Albany, NY, State University of New York Press: 11–38.

Miller, C.G. and D.W. Miller (2011). 'The real world failure of evidence-based medicine.' *International Journal of Person Centered Medicine* 1(2): 295–300.

Miller, P. (1991). 'Accounting and objectivity: The invention of calculating selves and calculable spaces.' *Annals of Scholarship* 8(3/4): 61–86.

Miller, P. and N. Rose (2008). *Governing the Present: Administering Social and Personal Life*. Cambridge, Polity.

Miller, W. (1998). *The Anatomy of Disgust*. Cambridge, MA, Harvard University Press.

Mishel, M.H. (1981). 'The measurement of uncertainty in illness.' *Nursing Research* 30(5): 258–263.

Moody, K. (2011). 'Capitalist care: Will the Coalition government's "reforms" move the NHS further toward a US-style healthcare market?' *Capital and Class* 35(3): 415–434.

Moore, W.E. and M.M. Tumin (1949). 'Some social functions of ignorance.' *American Sociological Review* 14: 787–795.

Moreton, A.P. (2005). 'Reflections on the Bundaberg hospital failure.' *Medical Journal of Australia* 183(6): 328–329.

Moreton-Robinson, A. (2009). 'Imagining the good indigenous citizen: Race war and the pathology of patriarchal white sovereignty.' *Cultural Studies Review* 15(2): 61–79.

Morse, K. (2001). 'Case in point? A parasuicide patient's recollections of being nursed: A discourse analysis.' *Contemporary Nurse* 10: 234–243.

Munhall, P.L. (1993). '"Unknowing": Toward another pattern of knowing.' *Nursing Outlook* 41: 125–128.

Myrick, F. (2005). 'Educating nurses for the knowledge economy.' *International Journal of Nursing Education Scholarship* 2(1): 20.

NACI (2012). *Statement on Seasonal Influenza Vaccine for 2012–2013*. National Advisory Committee on Immunization. *Canada Communicable Disease Report* 38, ACS-2. [Online], Available: www.phac-aspc.gc.ca/publicat/ccdr-rmtc/12vol38/acs-dcc-2/index-eng.php [accessed 28 January 2015].

Nozawa, S. (2012). 'Discourses of the coming: Ignorance, forgetting and prolepsis in Japanese life historiography.' *The Anthropology of Ignorance: An Ethnographic Approach*. C. High, A. Kelly and J. Mair. Houndsmill, UK, Palgrave Macmillan: 55–86.

Nelson, S. (2009). 'Historical amnesia and its consequences—the need to build histories of practice.' *Texto e Contexto-Enfermagen* 18(4): 781–787.

Nelson, S. (2012). 'The lost path to emancipatory practice: Towards a history of reflective practice in nursing.' *Nursing Philosophy* 13: 201–213.

Nelson, S. and A.M. Rafferty (2010). *Notes on Nightingale: The Influence and Legacy of a Nursing Icon*. Ithaca, NY, Cornell University Press.

NMC and GMC (2014). *Openness and Honesty When Things Go Wrong: The Professional Duty of Candour*. London, Nursing and Midwifery Council and General Medical Council.

O'Neill, S., T. Jones, D. Bennett and M. Lewis (2011). 'Nursing works: the application of lean thinking to nursing processes.' *Journal of Nursing Administration* 41: 556–552.

Osterholm, M.T., N.S. Kelley, A. Sommer, and E.A. Belongia (2012). 'Efficacy and effectiveness of influenza vaccines: A systematic review and meta-analysis.' *The Lancet Infectious Diseases* 12(1): 36–44.

Owen, N. (2012). '"Facts are sacred": *The Manchester Guardian* and colonial violence, 1930–1932.' *Journal of Modern History* 84(3): 643–678.

Paharia, N., K.D. Vohs, and R. Deshpandé (2013). 'Sweatshop labor is wrong unless the shoes are cute: Cognition can both hurt and help motivated moral reasoning.' *Organizational Behavior and Human Decision Processes* 121: 81–88.

Parker, J.M. (2004). 'Nursing on the medical ward.' *Nursing Inquiry* 11: 210–217.

Pearce, L. (2012). 'Triumph over taboos.' *Nursing Standard* 26(45): 24–25.

Pearson, A. (2010). 'Guest editorial: Evidence-based healthcare and qualitative research.' *Journal of Research in Nursing* 15(6): 489–493.

Pearson, A., R. Weichula, A. Court and C. Lockwood (2005). 'The JBI model of evidence-based healthcare.' *International Journal of Evidence-Based Healthcare* 2: 207–215.

Penrod, J. (2001). 'Refinement of the concept of uncertainty.' *Journal of Advanced Nursing* 34(2): 238–245.

Penrod, J. (2007). 'Living with uncertainty: Concept advancement.' *Journal of Advanced Nursing* 57(6): 658–667.

Perron, A., D. Holmes and C. Hamonet (2004). 'Capture, mortification, dépersonnalisation: La pratique infirmière en milieu correctionnel.' *Journal de réadaptation médicale* 24(4): 124–131.

Perron, A., C. Fluet and D. Holmes (2005). 'Agents of care and agents of the state: Bio-power and nursing practice.' *Journal of Advanced Nursing* 50(5): 536–544.

Perron, A., T. Rudge and M. Gagnon (2014). 'Towards an "ethics of discomfort" in nursing: Parrhesia as fearless speech.' *Philosophies and Practices of Emancipatory Nursing: Social Justice as Praxis.* P. Kagan, M. Smith and P. Chinn. New York, Routledge: 39–50.

Picco, E., R. Santoro, and L. Garrino (2010). 'Dealing with the patient's body in nursing: Nurses' ambiguous experience in clinical practice.' *Nursing Inquiry* 17(1): 39–46.

Pinney, J.A. (1979). 'The dark side of nursing: a twentieth century taboo.' *Nursing Mirror* 148(14): 14–20.

Poland, G.A. and S. Tucker (2012). 'Editorial: The nursing profession and patient safety and healthcare provider influenza immunization: The puzzling stance of the American Nursing Association.' *Vaccine* 30(10): 1753–1755.

Prasser, S. (2010). 'The Queensland Health Royal Commissions.' *Australian Journal of Public Administration* 69(1): 79–97.

Proctor, R.N. (2008). 'Agnotology: A missing term to describe the cultural production of ignorance (and its study).' *Agnotology: The Making and Unmaking of Ignorance.* R.N. Proctor and L. Schiebinger.Stanford, CA, Stanford University Press: 1–33.

Proctor, R.N. and L. Schiebinger (2008). *Agnotology: The Making and Unmaking of Ignorance.* Stanford, CA, Stanford University Press.

Puzan, E. (2003). 'The unbearable whiteness of being (in nursing).' *Nursing Inquiry* 10(3): 193–200.

Quested, B. (2010). 'Betwixt and between nothingness: Abjection and blood stem cell transplant.' *Abjectly Boundless: Boundaries, Bodies and Health Work.* T. Rudge and D. Holmes. Farnham, UK, Ashgate: 117–132.

Quested, B. and T. Rudge (2001). 'Procedure manuals and textually mediated death.' *Nursing Inquiry* 8(4): 264–272.

Quinn, M. (2011). 'Committing (to) ignorance: On method, myth, and pedagogy with Jacques Rancière.' *Epistemologies of Ignorance in Education.* E. Malewski and N. Jaramillo. Charlotte, NC, Information Age Publishers: 31–52.

Racine, L. (2003). 'Implementing a postcolonial feminist perspective in nursing research related to non-western populations.' *Nursing Inquiry* 10(2): 91–102.

Radder, H. (2010). *The Commodification of Academic Research: Science and the Modern University.* Pittsburgh, PA, University of Pittsburgh Press.

Rafferty, A.M. (1995). 'Art, science and social science in nursing: Occupational origins and disciplinary identity.' *Nursing Inquiry* 2: 141–148.

Rafferty, A.M. (1996). *The Politics of Nursing Knowledge.* London, Routledge.

Rafferty, A.M., N. Allcock and J. Lathlean (1996). 'The theory/practice "gap": taking issue with the issue.' *Journal of Advanced Nursing* 23(4): 685–691.

Ramsden, I. (1990). 'Cultural safety.' *New Zealand Nursing Journal Kai Tiaki* 83(11): 18–19.

Rankin, J. (2009). 'The nurse project: an analysis for nurses to take back our work.' *Nursing Inquiry* 16(4): 275–286.

Rauen, C.A., M. Chulay, E. Bridges, R.M. Vollman and R. Arbour (2008). 'Seven evidence-based practice habits: Putting some sacred cows out to pasture.' *Critical Care Nurse* 28(2): 98–123.

Ravetz, J.R. (1993). 'The sin of science. Ignorance of ignorance.' *Knowledge: Creation, Diffusion, Utilization* 15(2):157–165.

Rawls, J. (1971). *A Theory of Justice.* Cambridge, MA, Belknap Press.

Rayner, S. (2012). 'Uncomfortable knowledge: The social construction of ignorance in science and environmental policy discourses.' *Economy and Society* 41(1): 107–125.

Reed, P.G. and N.B.C. Shearer (2012). *Perspectives on Nursing Theory* (6th edn). Philadelphia, PA, Lippincott, Williams and Wilkins.

Reith, G. (2004). 'Uncertain times: The notion of "risk" and the development of modernity.' *Time and Society* 13(2/3): 383–402.

Rishel, T. (2011). 'Student suicide: The relevance (and luxury) of ignorance.' *Epistemologies of Ignorance in Education.* E. Malewski and N. Jaramillo. Charlotte, NC, Information Age Publishers: 167–185.

Ritchie, L. (2013). 'Photographs of the ageing body in a nursing journal: A profession's response.' *Nursing Inquiry* 20(2): 101–110.

Robert Wood Johnson Foundation (2010). 'Groundbreaking new survey finds that diverse opinion leaders say nurses should have more influence on health systems and services.' January 19. [Online], Available: www.rwjf.org/en/about-rwjf/newsroom/newsroom-content/2010/01/groundbreaking-new-survey-finds-that-diverse-opinion-leaders-say.html [16 Dec 2014].

Roberts, J. (2012). 'Organizational ignorance: towards a managerial perspective on the unknown.' *Management Learning* 44(3): 215–236.

Roberts, J. and J. Armitage (2008). 'The ignorance economy.' *Prometheus* 26(4): 335–354.

Robertson-Malt, S. (1998). 'Tolerance in ambiguity: Supporting the donor family.' *Nursing Inquiry* 5(3), 194–196.

Robinson, K. and B. Vaughan (1992). *Knowledge for Nursing Practice.* Oxford, Butterworth Heinemann.

Roderick, A. (2010). 'Dirty nursing: Containment and infection control practices.' *Abjectly Boundless: Boundaries, Bodies and Health Work.* T. Rudge and D. Holmes. Farnham, UK, Ashgate: 239–251.

Rose, N. (2005). 'Will biomedicine transform society? The political, economic, social and personal impact of medical advances in the twenty first century.' Clifford Barclay Lecture, 2 February.London School of Economics and Political Science.

Rose, N. (2007). *The Politics of Life Itself.* Princeton, NJ, Princeton University Press.

Ruckert, A. (2013). 'Global health governance after the financial crisis: making health equity matter.' *Canadian Foreign Policy Journal* 19(3): 340–353.

Rudge, T. (1999). 'Situating wound management: Technoscience, dressings and "other" skins.' *Nursing Inquiry* 6: 167–177.

Rudge, T. (2003). 'Words are powerful tools: discourse analytic explanations of nursing practice.' *Advanced Qualitative Nursing Research.* J. Latimer. Oxford, Blackwell Science: 151–181.

Rudge, T. (2009). 'Beyond caring? Discounting the differently known body.' *The Unknown/Known Body.* J. Latimer and M. Schillmeier. London, Sociological Review Monographs Remembering Elites Series: 233–248.

Rudge, T. (2011). 'The "well-run" system and its antimonies.' *Nursing Philosophy* 12: 167–176.

Rudge, T. (2013). 'Desiring productivity: nary a wasted moment, never a missed step!' *Nursing Philosophy* 14(3): 201–211.

Rudge, T. (2015). 'Julia Kristeva: Abjection, embodiment and boundaries.' *Handbook of Social Theory.* F. Collyer. London, Palgrave Macmillan.

Rudge, T. and D. Holmes (2010). *Abjectly Boundless: Boundaries, Bodies and Health Work*. Farnham, UK, Ashgate.

Rudge, T., A. Perron and D. Holmes (2011). 'The rise of practice development with/in reformed bureaucracy: Discourse, power, and the government of nursing.' *Journal of Nursing Management* 19: 837–844.

Sackett, D.L. (1989). 'Rules of evidence and clinical recommendations on the use of antithrombotic agents.' *Chest* 95: 2–4.

Sackett, D.L., W.M.C. Rosenberg, J.A.M. Gray, R.B. Haynes and W.S. Richardson (1996). 'Evidence based medicine: What it is and what it isn't.' *British Medical Journal* 312: 71–72.

Said, E.W. (2003). *Orientalism*. Harmondsworth, UK, Penguin.

Saltzberg, C.W. (2002). 'Nursing students' uncertainty experiences and epistemological perspectives.' PhD thesis, Ithaca, NY, Cornell University.

Schabas, R. and N. Rau (2015). 'Are we taking the flu (shot) too seriously?' *The Globe and Mail* January 24. [Online], Available: www.theglobeandmail.com/globe-debate/are-we-taking-the-flu-shot-too-seriously/article22602526/ [accessee 25 January 2015].

Schely-Newman, E. (2011). 'Eradicating ignorance: A gendered literacy campaign.' *Nashim: A Journal of Jewish Women's Studies and Gender Issues* 22: 15–31.

van Schendel, W. (2002). 'Geographies of knowing, geographies of ignorance: Jumping scale in South East Asia.' *Environment and Planning D: Society and Space* 20: 647–668.

Schick Makaroff, K., L. Shields and A. Molzahn (2013). 'Stories of chronic kidney disease: Listening for the unsayable.' *Journal of Advanced Nursing* 69(12): 2644–2653.

Schiebinger, L. (2008). 'West Indian abortifacients and the making of ignorance.' *Agnotology: The Making and Unmaking of Ignorance*. R.N. Proctor and L. Schiebinger. Stanford, CA: Stanford University Press: 149–162.

Schmied, V. and D. Lupton (2010). 'Blurring the boundaries: Breastfeeding and maternal subjectivity.' *Abjectly Boundless: Boundaries, Bodies and Health Work*. T. Rudge and D. Holmes. Farnham, UK, Ashgate: 15–31.

Schön, D.A. (1988). 'From technical rationality to reflection in action.' *Professional Judgement: A Reader in Clinical Decision Making*. J. Dowie and A. Elstein. Cambridge, Cambridge University Press: 60–77.

Scott, I.A., P.J. Poole and S. Jayathissa (2008). 'Improving quality and safety of hospital care: A reappraisal and an agenda for clinically relevant reform.' *Internal Medicine Journal* 38: 44–55.

Sedgwick, E. (2008). *Epistemologies of the Closet* (2nd edn). Berkeley, CA, University of California Press.

Sheikh, M.A. (2011). 'Good data and intelligent government.' *New Directions for Intelligent Government in Canada*. F. Gorbet and A. Sharpe.Ottawa, Centre for the Study of Living Standards: 305–335.

Shribman, D. (2006). 'A shameful ignorance of history.' *Buffalo News* [Final Edition]. Buffalo, NY. 30 September: A7.

Siddle, D.J. (1992). 'Urbanisation, population mobility and the evolution of cultural prejudice: Some speculations on the geography of ignorance and the growth of national identity.' *Geografiska Annaler, Series B, Human Geography* 74(3): 155–166.

Simon, D. (1998). 'Rethinking (post)modernism, postcolonialism, and posttradition alism: South–North perspectives.' *Environment and Planning D: Society and Space* 16: 219–245.

Simonsen, L., T.A. Reichert, C. Viboud, W.C. Blackwelder, R.J. Taylor and M.A. Miller (2005). 'Impact of influenza vaccination on seasonal mortality in the US elderly population.' *Archives of Internal Medicine* 165(3): 265–272.

Sinclair, M. (2000). *The Report of the Manitoba Pediatric Cardiac Surgery Inquest: An Inquiry into Twelve Deaths at the Winnipeg Health Sciences Centre in 1994.* Winnipeg, Provincial Court of Manitoba.

Singh, J. (2014). 'The ideological roots of Stephen Harper's vendetta against sociology.' *The Toronto Star* August 26. [Online], Available: www.thestar.com/opinion/comm entary/2014/08/26/the_ideological_roots_of_stephen_harpers_vendetta_against_socio logy.html [accessed 27 January 2015].

Skowronski, D.M., C. Chambers, S. Sabaiduc, G. De Serres, J.A. Dickinson, A.L. Winter et al. (2015). 'Interim estimates of 2014/15 vaccine effectiveness against influenza A(H3N2) from Canada's Sentinel Physician Surveillance Network, January 2015.' *Euro Surveillance* 20(4), 21022. [Online], Available: www.euro surveillance.org/ViewArticle.aspx?ArticleId=21022 [accessed 1 February 2015].

Slovic, P., M.L. Finucane, E. Peters and D.G. MacGregor (2004). 'Risk as analysis and risk as feelings: Some thoughts about affect, reason, risk, and rationality.' *Risk Analysis* 24: 311–322.

Smith, R. (1992). 'The ethics of ignorance.' *Journal of Medical Ethics* 18: 117–118, 134.

Smith, R. (2005). 'Medical journals are an extension of the marketing arm of pharmaceutical companies.' *PLoS Med* 2(5): e138.

Smithson, M. (1985). 'Toward a social theory of ignorance.' *Journal for the Theory of Social Behaviour* 15(2): 151–172.

Smithson, M. (1989). *Ignorance and Uncertainty: Emerging Paradigms* (Cognitive Science Series). New York, Springer Verlag.

Smithson, M. (2008). 'Social theories of ignorance.' *Agnotology: The Making and Unmaking of Ignorance.* R.N. Proctor and L. Schiebinger. Stanford, CA, Stanford University Press: 209–229.

Snyder-Halpern, R., S. Corcoran-Perry and S. Narayan (2001). 'Developing clinical practice environments supporting the knowledge work of nurses.' *Computers in Nursing* 19(1): 17–23.

Sokal, A.D. (2006). 'Pseudoscience and postmodernism: Antagonists or fellow travelers?' *Archaeological Fantasies: How Pseudoarchaeology Misrepresents the Past and Misleads the Public.* G. Fagan.New York, Routledge: 286–361.

Sokal, A.D. and J. Bricmont (1998). *Fashionable Nonsense: Postmodern Intellectuals' Abuse of Science.* New York, Picador.

Sorenson, O. (2003). 'Social networks and industrial geography.' *Journal of Evolutionary Economics* 13: 513–527.

Sorrell Dinkins, C. (2011). 'Ethics: Beyond patient care: Practicing empathy in the workplace.' *OJIN: The Online Journal of Issues in Nursing* 16(2).

Stenhouse, J. (2005). 'Imperialism, atheism, and race: Charles Southwell, old corruption and the Maori.' *Journal of British Studies* 44(4): 754–774.

Strathern, M. (2000). *Audit Cultures: Anthropological Studies in Accountability, Ethics and the Academy.* London, Routledge.

Street, A. (1990). *Nursing Practice: High, Hard Ground, Messy Swamps and the Pathways in Between.* Geelong, VIC, Deakin University Press.

Sullivan, P.L. (2009). 'Influenza vaccination in healthcare workers: Should it be mandatory?' *OJIN: The Online Journal of Issues in Nursing* 15(1).

Sullivan, S. and N. Tuana (Eds) (2007). *Race and Epistemologies of Ignorance*. Albany, NY: SUNY Press.

Swan, E. (2010). 'States of white ignorance, and audit masculinity in English higher education.' *Social Politics* 17(4): 477–506.

Swendson, C. and C. Windsor (1996). 'Rethinking cultural sensitivity.' *Nursing Inquiry* 3: 3–10.

Takala, J. (1999). 'The right to genetic ignorance.' *Bioethics*, 13(3/4): 288–293.

Tantchou, J. C. (2014). 'Blurring boundaries: Structural constraints, space, tools, and agency in an operating theater.' *Science, Technology and Human Values* 39(3): 336–373.

Teasdale, K. and G. Kent (1995). 'The use of deception in nursing.' *Journal of Medical Ethics* 21:77–81.

Thomas, RE., T. Jefferson and T.J. Lasserson (2013). 'Influenza vaccination for healthcare workers who care for people aged 60 or older living in long-term care institutions.' *Cochrane Database of Systematic Reviews* 2013(7): CD005187. DOI: 10.1002/14651858.CD005187.pub4.

Thompson, C. and D. Dowding (2001). 'Responding to uncertainty in nursing practice.' *International Journal of Nursing Studies* 38: 609–615.

Thrift, N. (2004). 'Remembering the technological unconscious by foregrounding knowledges of position.' *Environment and Planning: Society and Space* 22: 175–190.

Thurlow, C. and A. Jaworski (2012). 'Elite mobilities: the semiotic landscapes of luxury and privilege.' *Social Semiotics* 22(4): 487–516.

Torjesen, I. (2014). 'Tamiflu purchase worth £49m will go ahead, government says.' *British Medical Journal* 348: g2761.

Toronto, C.E. and S.M. Mullaney (2010). 'Registered nurses and influenza vaccination. An integrative review.' *American Association of Occupational Health Nurses Journal* 58(11): 463–471.

Townley, C. (2006). 'Toward a revaluation of ignorance.' *Hypatia* 21: 37–55.

Townley, C. (2011). *A Defense of Ignorance: Its Value for Knowers and Roles in Feminist and Social Epistemologies*. Lanham, MD, Lexington Books.

Traynor, M. (2014). 'Caring after Francis: Moral failure in nursing reconsidered.' *Journal of Research in Nursing* 19(7/8): 546–556.

Tuana, N. (2006). 'The speculum of ignorance: The women's health movement and epistemologies of ignorance.' *Hypatia* 21(3): 1–19.

Tuana, N. (2008). 'Coming to understand: Orgasm and the epistemology of ignorance.' *Agnotology: The Making and Unmaking of Ignorance*. R.N. Proctor and L. Schiebinger. Stanford, CA, Stanford University Press: 108–145.

Tuckett, A. (1998). '"Bending the truth": Professionals' narratives about lying and deception in nursing practice.' *International Journal of Nursing Studies* 35: 292–302.

Tuckett, A. (2004). 'Truth-telling in clinical practice and the arguments for and against: A review of the literature.' *Nursing Ethics* 11(5): 500–513.

Ungar, S. (2008). 'Ignorance as an under-identified social problem.' *British Journal of Sociology* 59(2): 301–326.

Urban, A.-M. (2014). 'Taken for granted: Normalizing nurses' work in hospitals.' *Nursing Inquiry* 21(1): 69–78.

US Government (1993). *Policy concerning homosexuality in the armed forces*. Pub. L. 103–160, USC 10, §654(a)(15). Nov 30 [Online], Available: http://www.gpo.gov/fdsys/pkg/USCODE-2010-title10/pdf/USCODE-2010-title10-subtitleA-partII-chap37-sec654.pdf [accessed 14 December 2014].

Vaismoradi, M., M. Salsali and F. Ahmadi (2010). 'Nurses' experiences of uncertainty in clinical practice: A descriptive study.' *Journal of Advanced Nursing* 67(5): 991–999.

Van Herk, K.A., D. Smith and C. Andrew. (2011). 'Examining our privileges and oppressions: Incorporating an intersectionality paradigm into nursing.' *Nursing Inquiry* 18(1): 29–39.

Varenne, H. (2009). 'Conclusion: The powers of ignorance: On finding out what to do next.' *Critical Studies in Education* 50: 337–343.

Vaughan, D. (1999). 'The dark side of organizations: mistake, misconduct, and disaster.' *Annual Review of Sociology* 25: 271–305.

Vitebsky, P. (1993). 'Is death the same everywhere? Contexts of knowing and doubting.' *An Anthropological Critique of Development: The Growth of Ignorance.* M. Hobart. London, Routledge: 100–115.

Walter, T. (1991). 'Modern death: Taboo or not taboo?' *Sociology* 25(2): 293–310.

Wang, L.Y., M. Davis, L. Robin, J. Collins, K. Coyle and E. Baumler, (2000). 'Economic evaluation of safer choices: A school-based human immunodeficiency virus, other sexually transmitted diseases, and pregnancy prevention program'. *Archives of Pediatric and Adolescent Medicine* 154(10): 1017–1024.

Warner, J.C. (2012). 'Overcoming barriers to influenza vaccination.' *Nursing Times* 108(37): 25–27.

Waska, R. (2011). *Moments of Uncertainty in Therapeutic Practice. Interpreting Within the Matrix of Projective Identification, Countertransference, and Enactment.* New York, Columbia University Press.

White, J. (1995). 'Patterns of knowing: review, critique, and update.' *Advances in Nursing Science* 17(4): 73–86.

WHO (2014). *Fact sheet no. 211. Influenza (Seasonal).* Geneva, World Health Organization.

Wolloch, N. (2007). '"Facts or conjectures": Antoine-Yves Gouget's historiography.' *Journal of the History of Ideas* 68(3): 429–449.

Wylie, A. (2008). 'Mapping ignorance in archeology: The advantages of historical hindsight.' *Agnotology: The Making and Unmaking of Ignorance.* R.N. Proctor and L. Schiebinger. Stanford, CA, Stanford University Press: 183–205.

Yancy, G. (2008). *Black Bodies, White Gazes: The Continuing Significance of Race.* Lanham, MD, Rowman and Littlefield.

Zuger, A. (1997). 'New way of doctoring: By the book.' *The New York Times* December 16. [Online], Available: www.nytimes.com/1997/12/16/science/new-way-of-doctoring-by-the-book.html [accessed 1 December 2014].

Index